Home Care Advances

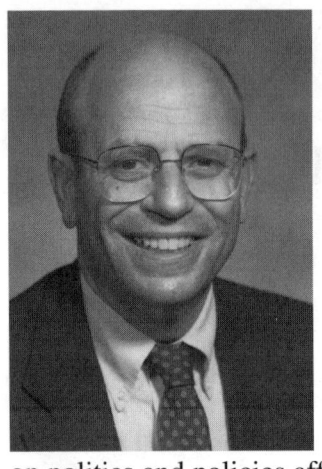
Robert H. Binstock, Ph.D., is professor of Aging, Health, and Society at Case Western Reserve University. A former president of the Gerontological Society of America, he has served as director of a White House Task Force on Older Americans for President Lyndon B. Johnson and as chairman and member of a number of advisory panels to the federal government, state and local governments, and foundations. He is immediate past chair of the Gerontological Health Section of the American Public Health Association. Professor Binstock is the author of nearly 200 publications on politics and policies affecting aging. His 20 books include *The Future of Long-term Care: Social and Policy Issues,* coedited with Leighton E. Cluff and Otto von Mering (Johns Hopkins University Press, 1996), and four editions of the *Handbook of Aging and the Social Sciences,* the most recent coedited with Linda K. George (Academic Press, 1996). He has received numerous honors and awards in the field of gerontology.

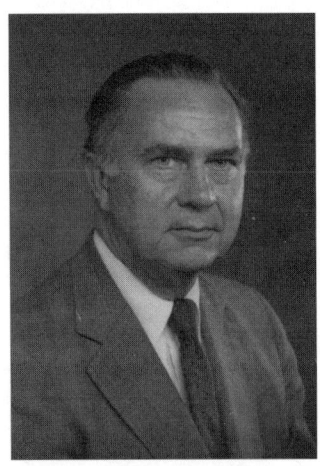
Leighton E. Cluff, M.D., is immediate past president and trustee emeritus of the Robert Wood Johnson Foundation. He is presently Professor Emeritus at the University of Florida, where he serves as member of the University of Florida Health Science Board of Overseers, Advisor to the University Center on Gerontology, member of the board of the Institute of Child Health Policy, and member of the board of the Geriatric Research and Education Center (Department of Veterans Affairs–Gainesville). He is also a member of the board of the Florida Foundation on Active Aging, and has served as chair of the Governor's and Legislature's Working Group on Health Care Reform for Florida (1990–1991). He is a master of the American College of Physicians. Dr. Cluff has published more than 200 scholarly articles and many book chapters. Among his books are *Helping Shape America's Health Care* (Robert Wood Johnson Foundation, 1989) and *The Future of Long-term Care: Social and Policy Issues,* coedited with Robert H. Binstock and Otto von Mering (Johns Hopkins University Press, 1996).

Home Care Advances

ESSENTIAL RESEARCH AND POLICY ISSUES

Robert H. Binstock, PhD
Leighton E. Cluff, MD
Editors

 SPRINGER PUBLISHING COMPANY

Copyright © 2000 by Springer Publishing Company, Inc.

All rights reserved.

No part of this publication may be reproduced, stored in a retrieval system, or transmitted in any form or by any means, electronic, mechanical, photocopying, recording, or otherwise, without the prior permission of Springer Publishing Company, Inc.

Springer Publishing Company, Inc.
536 Broadway
New York, NY   10012-3955

Acquisitions Editor: Bill Tucker
Production Editor: Jeanne Libby
Cover design by James Scotto-Lavino

00 01 02 03 04 / 5 4 3 2 1

Library of Congress Cataloging-in-Publication Data

Home care advances : essential research and policy issues / Robert H. Binstock and Leighton E. Cluff, editors.
    p.   cm.
   Includes bibliographical references and index.
   ISBN 0-8261-1304-4
    1. Aged—Home care—United States.   2. Aged—Home care—Social aspects—United States.   3. Aged—Long-term care—United States.   4. Home care services—Research—United States.   I. Binstock, Robert H.   II. Cluff, Leighton E.

RA645.35 .H645 2000
362.1'9897—dc21

                                                               99-054282

Printed in the United States of America

Contents

Contributors	*vii*
Preface	*ix*

Section One: Overview

1. **Issues and Challenges in Home Care** — 3
   Robert H. Binstock and Leighton E. Cluff
2. **The Changing Health and Social Environments of Home Care** — 35
   Donna M. Cox and Marcia G. Ory

Section Two: The Provision of Home Care

3. **The Use of Technology in Home Care** — 59
   Leighton E. Cluff and Patricia Flatley Brennan
4. **Families and Paid Workers: The Complexities of Home Care Roles** — 78
   Baila Miller
5. **Hospice: End-of-Life Care at Home** — 101
   Patrice C. Moore and Robert H. McCollough
6. **Home Care as a Business** — 117
   Robert D. Hutson

Section Three: Financing, Auspices, and Quality of Care

7. **Issues in Understanding Resource Consumption in Publicly Funded Home Care** — 137
   Richard H. Fortinsky and Elizabeth A. Madigan
8. **Shaping Home Care by Measuring Outcomes** — 163
   Peter W. Shaughnessy
9. **Testing Home Care as a Managed Care Intervention** — 191
   Susan L. Hughes and Frances M. Weaver
10. **Assuring Quality in Care at Home** — 207
    Rosalie A. Kane

Section Four: The Issues and Challenges Ahead

11. **The Uncertain Future of Home Care** — 239
    Carroll L. Estes

Index — *257*

Contributors

Patricia Flateley Brennan, Ph.D.
School of Nursing and College of Engineering
University of Wisconsin-Madison
Madison, WI

Donna M. Cox, Ph.D.
Department of Health Science
Towson State University
Towson, MD

Carroll L. Estes, Ph.D.
Institute for Health and Aging
University of California at San Francisco
San Francisco, CA

Richard H. Fortinsky, Ph.D.
Center on Aging
University of Connecticut
Farmington, CT

Susan L. Hughes, D.S.W.
Prevention Research Center
School of Public Health
University of Illinois—Chicago
Chicago, IL

Robert D. Hutson
Hutson Industries, Inc.
Gainesville, FL

Rosalie A. Kane, D.S.W.
Division for Health Services Research and Policy
School of Public Health
University of Minnesota
Minneapolis, MN

Elizabeth A. Madigan, Ph.D.
Bolton School of Nursing
Case Western Reserve University
Cleveland, OH

Robert McCollough, M.D.
Hospice of North Central Florida
Gainesville, FL

Baila Miller, Ph.D.
Mandel School of Applied Social Sciences
Case Western Reserve University
Cleveland, OH

Patrice C. Moore, M.S.N., A.R.N.P.
Hospice of North Central Florida
Gainesville, FL

Marcia G. Ory, Ph.D.
Social Science Research
    Division
National Institute on Aging
Bethesda, MD

Peter W. Shaughnessy, Ph.D.
Center for Health Services Research
University of Colorado Health
    Sciences Center
Denver, CO

Frances M. Weaver, Ph.D.
Institute for Health Services
    Research and Policy Studies
Northwestern University
Evanston, IL

Preface

Beginning in 1992, the University of Florida held the first of five National Health Care Forums with support from the Robert Wood Johnson Foundation. At the first forum on long-term care, Robert H. Binstock was a keynote speaker. He, Leighton E. Cluff, and Otto von Mering edited a book based on that forum, entitled *Long-term Care: Social and Policy Issues,* published by the Johns Hopkins University Press in 1996. In following years forums were held on raising children; abuse of children, spouses, and the elderly; physician-assisted death; and home care. This book, *Home Care Advances: Essential Research and Policy Issues,* is the second major publication resulting from these National Health Care Forums. Many nationally recognized experts have contributed to these forums, and their contributions are most appreciated.

The University of Florida's Forum on Home Care was initiated in 1996 by Leighton Cluff with support from the Robert Wood Johnson Foundation. David Challoner, vice president for Health Affairs, University of Florida, and Paul Metz, director of the Shands Hospital of the University of Florida, were supportive of this undertaking. Professor Raymond Coward, working with Cluff, had responsibility for organizing and administering a series of seminars on home care. National experts on this topic were invited to make presentations and meet with various faculty members involved in programs on aging at the university. The plan for this series of visits also included the publication of the visitors' papers in a book. Subsequently, Professor Coward accepted a position at the University of New Hampshire, and unforeseen circumstances prevented preparation of the manuscripts for publication.

In 1998 Dr. Marcia G. Ory of the National Institute on Aging encouraged Leighton Cluff to ask the contributors to *update* their manuscripts for publication of a book on home care. All contributors agreed, and their updated manuscripts (in some cases with the participation of coauthors) form most of the substance of this book, along with three additional chapters. Marcia Ory's contribution to this effort was significant and is deeply appreciated.

Robert Binstock did not contribute to the Seminars on Home Care, but he and Leighton Cluff had previously worked effectively together in the development and editing of the book *Long-term Care: Social and Policy Issues*. Therefore, in late 1998, he agreed to work with Cluff in editing this volume. As the updated papers came in, Binstock joined Cluff in the substantial editorial work on the manuscripts, and in the authorship of the opening chapter.

We appreciate the interest and encouragement provided by Ursula Springer and her agreement to have this book published by the Springer Publishing Company.

OVERVIEW OF THE VOLUME

The opening section of this book provides an introductory landscape of home care in the United States and how it has evolved to the present day. In chapter 1, the editors define and describe home care and present a brief picture of the contemporary need for it; trace the evolution of public policies that have enabled paid home care services to be used extensively by patients and their families; examine the substantial role of families in providing care and their efforts to pay for it, including the role played by private insurance and the phenomenon of Medicaid "estate planning"; and highlight a series of major issues and challenges concerning the provision of home care as we begin the 21st century. In chapter 2, Donna M. Cox and Marcia G. Ory discuss home care in the context of changing health and social environments. They review the conditions of illness, disability, and functional limitations that lead people to need long-term care in general, and home care in particular. Cox and Ory then examine the changing home care industry and home care use and trends; explicate the nature of home care, including its goals and the models through which it is provided; analyze changes in the concept of home care; and offer a substantial agenda of research for future refinements in the delivery of home care.

The second section of the volume sets forth a series of perspectives on the provision of home care. The use of technology in home care, particularly high-tech medical care and computer and other communication technologies, is presented by Leighton E. Cluff and Patricia Flatley Brennan in chapter 3. They also analyze the key roles that need to be played by health professionals and caring families when high-tech medical care is provided. They conclude with a series of societal concerns that arise from the use of technology in home care—economic issues, ethical and legal issues, and challenges to public policy.

In chapter 4, Baila Miller delineates issues that arise when care is provided to the same individual both by unpaid family members and by paid professionals and paraprofessionals. She begins by focusing on the roles that family members play as informal caregivers, then the roles played by formal service providers, and the ways in which family and cultural contexts can shape these roles. Building on this foundation, Miller explores the complex relations between family and paid caregivers and lays out some policy issues that arise from them.

Hospice as a form of home care for the terminally ill is the subject of chapter 5, by Patrice C. Moore and Robert H. McCollough. They begin with an explication of the unique concept of hospice care and its introduction to the United States from England. They then trace the evolution of hospice from a largely voluntary effort to a well-funded program under Medicare, describing the settings for care (predominantly home care), its recipients, and the range and nature of services provided. Moore and McCollough conclude by setting forth issues and challenges that will shape the future of hospice and its role within the health care arena.

This section concludes with chapter 6, which looks at the provision of home care from a business perspective. The author, Robert D. Hutson, has been in the field of health care management since 1976, and has managed home health agencies from 1982 to 1997. Drawing on his considerable experience, he presents a picture of the various segments of the home care business—Medicare-certified home health, private duty services, durable medical equipment, home infusion or intravenous therapy, fetal monitoring at home, specialty blood products, and various "carve outs" through which patients with a particular disease or condition are targeted through services and products that are particularly relevant to them (e.g., biotech drugs). Hutson then sets forth his views on priority administrative challenges facing the industry and managed care's role in home care. Finally, he offers various strategies for success.

Four chapters make up the third section of the volume, which deals with various aspects of financing, auspices, and quality in home care. The rapid growth of public funding for home care during the 1990s brought a great deal of attention to the factors that account for the increase in costs, in addition to the growth of the population needing care. In chapter 7, Richard H. Fortinsky and Elizabeth A. Madigan explore what is known and not known about resource consumption in publicly funded home care. They begin with a review of the government-established eligibility criteria that drive the demand for public funding of home care. They then present the state of the art in measuring resource consumption by reviewing the various units of analysis that have been used—the number of home care visits, lengths of visits, episodes of home care, and staff mix. Next, they examine various predictors of resource consumption—at the patient level, the agency level, and the system level. Fortinsky and Madigan also analyze the relationships between resource consumption and patient outcomes and conclude by posing a series of additional questions that need to be investigated.

Resource consumption and patient outcomes in home care is also the subject of chapter 8. Peter W. Shaughnessy presents a line of ongoing research on costs, auspices, and outcomes in home care that has been developed at the Center for Health Services Research, University of Colorado Health Sciences Center. He illustrates the center's approach by summarizing a study of costs and patient outcomes that compared home care provided under managed care with care provided through the traditional fee-for-service system, and indicated that there is reason to be concerned about quality of home care provided through managed care. Shaughnessy lays out the Center's approach and results from work on measuring outcomes and implementing an outcome-based quality improvement system. Finally, he offers an approach for simultaneous evaluation of home care costs and outcomes.

A different approach to the issue of costs and auspices is undertaken in chapter 9. Susan L. Hughes and Frances M. Weaver report on several demonstration studies of the cost-effectiveness of innovative hospital-based home care management models undertaken in the Chicago area. High-risk patients were targeted for ongoing primary care management in home care, including direct "hands on" involvement of the home care physician or the explicit use of condition-specific home care protocols that were developed jointly by home care staff and relevant physician specialists. The first of these studies demonstrated cost savings through this approach; two other studies, with slightly varied approaches, are ongoing.

The central focus of the last chapter in section 3 is quality assurance. In chapter 10, Rosalie A. Kane offers a comprehensive discussion of the topic, starting with an analysis of the methods available for assessing quality in home care. Next, she sets forth an ideal model of quality assurance practices, as well as the approaches through which they can be implemented—regulatory, consumer-centered, market/systemic, educational, and provider-initiated. After discussing a number of unresolved issues in quality assurance, she concludes by laying out a substantial future agenda, including conceptual challenges, research questions, and possible demonstration projects and major initiatives.

The final section of the volume consists of a chapter by Carroll L. Estes, which examines the past and likely future of home care from a public policy perspective. Estes analyzes the impact of what she sees as five "waves of change" in home care, from 1978 through the enactment of the Balanced Budget Act of 1997 which provided for reductions in Medicare payments for home health services. She examines a series of contemporary issues likely to affect the future of home care—managed care and the "free rider" problem, the problem of the "no care zone," and a variety of political and economic trends. Estes concludes with a set of central principles to guide home care policies in the years immediately ahead.

SECTION ONE

OVERVIEW

CHAPTER 1

Issues and Challenges in Home Care

Robert H. Binstock
Leighton E. Cluff

This volume examines contemporary and future issues and challenges concerning home health care in the United States for people who are ill and disabled, including those who need continuing care after they are released from hospitals, nursing homes, and other health care institutions. Home care comprises a wide variety of services, including those provided by the affected person, family, friends, and various community support groups, as well as by professionals who are part of organized systems for the provision of home care.

Home health care is hardly a new phenomenon. From the beginning of human existence people have received care where they live. Each and every person, at one time or another, has been cared for in the home—infants, children, adolescents, and adults suffering from acute or chronic illnesses; persons of all ages who are functionally limited in their activities of daily living because of frailty and disability; and those who are terminally ill.

From the American colonial period through the early decades of the 20th century, care of the ill in the United States was predominantly community-based rather than institutional. Although institutions for care of the poor began to develop around 1820, medical care—except for the poorest persons—still took place in the home (Cole, 1996). After the enactment of Social Security during the 1930s, even some of the poor were better able to remain in their own homes for care because of the income now available to them through retirement benefits and Old Age Assistance welfare payments.

In the first half of the 20th century, when there was little to do but feed, bathe, dress, and support the ill and disabled at home, specially trained or professional persons were rarely required. Relatively little consideration was given to visiting a doctor's office or clinic. The technologies available in physicians' offices, clinics, and hospitals—except for major surgical procedures—usually were available in the home, or could be carried in a "medical bag." Physicians, when needed, made "house calls." (Public health nurses and the Visiting Nurse Associations, however, did provide some professional and support services in the home, particularly for patients discharged from hospitals.)

Only in recent times has care in the home become more than that provided by families, friends, and community groups, occasionally supplemented by professional services. A number of factors have transformed the landscape of home health care.

Family and community structures have changed. In contemporary America family members are often geographically distant, and thus unable to provide care for each other. Far greater proportions of adult females, the traditional caregivers in home settings, are employed workers; for them, it is difficult, if not impossible, to care for a family member at home supplemented by only occasional professional medical and nursing services. Many family caregivers themselves are old and need some measure of supportive assistance. Although neighbors, friends, and religious organizations are sometimes able to help fill the void, an overall consequence has been increasing dependency on health professionals and other specially trained persons to provide such care.

In addition, home care became a more viable alternative to care in nursing homes and other institutions for the chronically ill and disabled as the federal and state governments began to provide reimbursement for home health services in the late 1960s following the enactment of Medicare and Medicaid. Today, reimbursements for home care that are provided through these two programs are the most rapidly growing sector of governmental expenditures for health care.

This introductory chapter provides an overview of home care in the United States and highlights major issues and challenges concerning its provision as we begin the 21st century. It begins with a brief picture of the contemporary need for home care. Next, it traces the evolution of public policies, particularly Medicare and Medicaid, that have enabled paid home care services to be used extensively by patients and their families. Then it examines the substantial role of families in providing care, arranging for care, the difficulties they face in paying for care out-of-pocket if Medicare and Medicaid reimbursement are not available to them, the part played by private insurance in paying for home care, and the phenomenon of Medicaid "estate planning" through which some individuals are able to have a program for the poor reimburse their care while avoiding the expenditure of their own assets to pay for care. Finally, it sets forth issues and challenges for the future that will be essential to address if home care is to be sufficient in quantity and quality in the decades ahead—the growth in demand for care, a possible decline in family caregiving, the potential applications of information technology, better orientation of health care professions to home care, and the need for greater public funding.

WHO NEEDS HOME CARE?

Individuals need and receive home care for a variety of reasons (in addition to relatively minor illnesses such as heavy colds, influenza, and other nonacute diseases that may confine a person to home for a short period). Subacute care and, often, rehabilitation are needed for patients who are discharged from hospitals to home, rather than to a skilled nursing facility. The highest volumes of such posthospital episodes of home care are for patients whose diagnosis-related groups (DRGs) during hospitalization are major joint and limb reattachment procedure (of lower extremity), heart failure and shock, specific cerebrovascular disorders (except transient ischemic attacks), simple pneumonia and pleurisy, chronic obstructive pulmonary disease, major small and large bowel procedures, hip and femur procedures (except major joint), and coronary bypass with cardiac catheterization (National Association for Home Care, 1997).

In addition, because of advances in medical technology, persons who are heavily dependent on technological support for their ongoing survival are now cared for in the home rather than in hospitals and other institutions (see chapter 3). As biomedical ethicist John Arras (1995) observed:

> [T]he high-tech home care industry has rapidly and relentlessly erased, for increasing numbers of families, the boundary between hospital and home, between the intensive care unit and the living room. More and more patients now receive in the privacy of their homes highly sophisticated medical treatments—such as ventilator therapy and artificial nutrition channeled through infusion pumps—that twenty years ago would have been available only in special care units. (p. xiii).

Home care is also provided for persons who need long-term care because they have chronic illnesses and disabilities that render them unable to carry on with normal activities of life in the absence of supportive care. The long-term care population consists of people who are unable to perform very basic activities of daily living (ADLs) or instrumental activities of daily living (IADLs), or some combination of them. ADLs are bathing, dressing, getting out of a chair or bed, toileting, and feeding oneself. IADLs include such activities as managing medications, managing money, shopping, preparing meals, light housework, using the phone, and traveling beyond a walking distance.

Among persons who need long-term care, 13.1 million are adults age 18 and older, and 0.4 million are children. Contrary to common perceptions, persons under the age of 65 constitute nearly half of the long-term care population. Fifty-five percent are age 65 and older, and 45% are younger (Feder, 1999).

The vast majority of the long-term care population needs home care; 88% reside in the community rather than in nursing homes. Among those in the community, there is substantial variation in functional limitations. Persons who are unable to perform independently three or more ADLs constitute 17%; those with one to two limitations in ADLs account for 24%; individuals who are limited only with respect to IADLs comprise 47% of the group (Feder, 1999).

PUBLIC POLICY AND THE EVOLUTION OF HOME CARE

As American medicine became more sophisticated in the middle decades of the 20th century, the predominance of the home as a setting for health care eroded for a while. But public policy resurrected the importance of home care. As Benjamin (1993) noted:

> With the emergence of modern scientific medicine and the hospitals in which it is practiced, the importance of home care waned as people sought care in hospitals and physician's offices. . . . Not until the marketing of private health insurance after World War II, and especially the passage of Medicare and Medicaid in 1965, was home care again to be considered a part of mainstream health care. (p. 129).

The enactment of the Medicare and Medicaid programs in 1965 (Titles 18 and 19 of the Social Security Act) made public financing available for professional home health services. This laid the foundation for increased use of formal, paid home care services, usually combined with informal care from family members and other unpaid caregivers (see chapter 4).

Initially, Medicaid and, to a more limited extent, Medicare financing fueled such a rapid expansion in nursing homes that these institutions became, in effect, a major alternative to home care (see Vladeck, 1980). Although the Medicare program included a home health benefit, use of it actually declined in the early 1970s (Callender & LaVor, 1975). Then, as Medicare and Medicaid spending for nursing homes mushroomed in these programs in the mid- to late 1970s, national and state politicians began to look to home care as a means of containing nursing home expenditures. Ironically, even as government financing had made nursing homes a widely available alternative to care in the home by families, now government sought to make home care a widely available alternative to nursing homes. (For an excellent discussion of the early political history of Medicare and Medicaid financing of long-term care, see Benjamin, 1993.)

In 1979 Congress authorized a major national demonstration project—the Channeling Demonstration—to explore the viability of expanded service coverage for home care, primarily as a means of reducing long-term care costs. The result was a multisite project, with case-managed services, which ran though 1985 and was subject to far greater evaluative methodological rigor than earlier efforts of this kind. The findings of the Channeling Demonstration (Kemper et al., 1988) should have been of no comfort to Congress. They indicated that home care was not a cost-effective alternative. As Weissert (1990) concluded, "That home care (home health, homemaker, daycare, and respite services and the like) is not a cost-effective substitute for nursing homes now appears to be a settled issue" (p. 42).

Nonetheless, politicians persisted in their belief that home care is more cost-effective than nursing home care. Moreover, they were convinced that most persons in need of care prefer to receive it in their own homes rather than in institutions (even though placement in a nursing home is often appropriate in terms of adequate care and safety as well as ongoing family life). Consequently, they have continually made public funding for home care more widely available at both the federal and the state levels. Medicare and Medicaid payments have fueled a proliferation of home care agencies, as was the case with nursing homes.

Medicare and Home Care

Medicare home health coverage was initially authorized only as a posthospital discharge benefit for a given number of days following the patient's discharge. The underlying notion of this benefit was that it would provide a cheaper alternative to extended hospital stays and reduce overall health care costs (Benjamin, 1993). Coverage was provided for nursing visits, services by medical social workers and physical, occupational, and speech therapists, medical supplies and equipment, and home health aides (providing nonmedical personal care and selected homemaker services). Required for this coverage was a "postacute" care plan provided by the patient's physician, who was expected to provide ongoing medical supervision. Although the 1965 legislation only provided Medicare home health coverage for persons age 65 and older, amendments in 1972 extended Medicare coverage, including home health, to younger persons who were receiving Social Security Disability Insurance and those with end-stage renal disease.

Expansions of Coverage

Medicare coverage for home health was expanded in the amendments to Medicare legislated in the Omnibus Reconciliation Act of 1980 (ORA80). The new law eliminated the requirement of a prior hospitalization and did away with the existing limit of 100 home health visits. It also eliminated deductibles and no longer required that for-profit home health agencies had to have state licenses (in those states that require them) in order to be reimbursed by Medicare.

Another important expansion of Medicare home care coverage occurred 2 years later. Hospice care for the terminally ill was authorized for reimbursement by the Tax Equity and Fiscal Responsibility Act of 1982 (see chapter 5). This extended home care coverage to an additional patient population, because 78% of hospice patients are cared for at home rather than in institutions (Haupt, 1998a).

Impact of Prospective Payment to Hospitals

The use of Medicare home health care accelerated in the mid-1980s following the shift of Medicare's reimbursements for hospital care from a retrospective basis to a prospective payment system (PPS). Under the previous reimbursement system hospitals had little incentive to discharge patients until they were well enough to go home and care for themselves, or until circumstances at home could accommodate the patients' limitations through care by the family.

With the implementation of PPS, Medicare began to pay hospitals a fixed sum for each inpatient's care, determined by which of hundreds of DRGs was applied to the diagnosis for each patient. Thus, hospitals had an incentive to discharge patients to home or a skilled nursing facility at an earlier stage of recovery than in the past, because they would receive the same amount from Medicare no matter how long the patients stayed in the hospital. These discharged patients often had substantial need for posthospital, subacute professional care, leading to an increased use of Medicare home health services. Medicare's expenditures for home care were augmented by these earlier discharges but, as shown in Figure 1.1, the increase was relatively small compared to the sharp growth in use of the home health benefit that began in the late 1980s.

Liberalization of Reimbursement Regulations

Considerable liberalization of home health coverage took place in 1989 because of a court order to the Health Care Financing Administration (HCFA), the federal agency that administers Medicare and Medicaid. A class action law suit in 1988 (*Duggan v. Bowen*) had challenged narrow interpretations that HCFA (and its fiscal intermediaries) had been making regarding reimbursement for part-time or intermittent care. The court

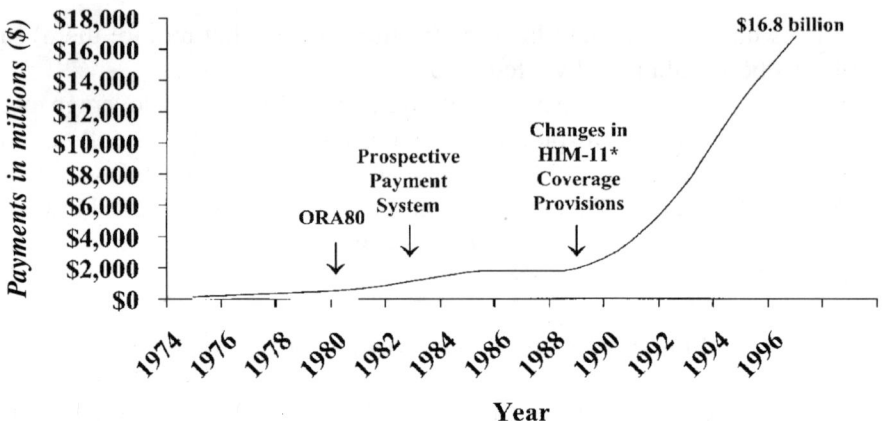

FIGURE 1.1 Medicare Home Health Agency Program payments: Calendar years 1974–1996.

*Medicare Health Insurance Manual-11.

Source: Health Care Financing Administration. (1998a).

ordered HCFA to reimburse for part-time care for as many as 7 days a week. In addition, HCFA's 1989 changes to its home health agency manual revised the interpretation of intermittent care to include reimbursement for skilled nursing and home health aide services up to 35 hours per week (see Bishop & Skawra, 1993).

Following the 1989 home health care revisions to HCFA's *Health Insurance Manual,* there was a dramatic growth in the volume of home care services and users covered by Medicare. As one might expect from the nature of the revisions, the most significant increase was in the number of home health service visits. From 1988 through 1996, visits increased by 602%, from 37.7 million to 264.8 million; similarly, the number of visits per 1,000 Medicare enrollees grew by 587%, from 1,144 to 7,857. The number of persons served increased 125%, from 1.6 million to 3.6 million; the user rate per 1,000 enrollees more than doubled, from 49 to 107 (Health Care Financing Administration, 1998a).

Accordingly, expenditures for Medicare home health care expanded at a dramatic pace. In the 1988–1996 period, payments to home health agencies increased by about 762%, from $1.9 billion to $16.8 billion. In 1996 these payments represented 10% of all Medicare fee-for-service payments (Health Care Financing Administration, 1998a).

Medicaid and Home Care

Medicaid also included a home health benefit when it was established in 1965 as a federal/state matching program to pay for medical assistance to designated categories of individuals and families with low incomes and meager financial resources. The program pays for home health care for persons eligible for skilled nursing services. Coverage for home care is not time limited. In contrast to the initial Medicare model, Medicaid is designed for long-term services to persons with chronic illnesses and disabilities, as well as acute care needs. About one third of Medicaid is spent on long-term care; of that, 27% is for home care, the balance for nursing home care (Health Care Financing Administration, 1998a).

The Omnibus Budget Reconciliation Act of 1981 extended Medicaid coverage by authorizing a special waiver program, which allows states to apply for federal Medicaid matching funds to provide a broader range of home- and community-based services (HCBS). The HCBS waiver program enables individuals to receive services that support IADLs—functions that are essential if the home is to remain viable as a residence. Eligibility for these supportive services requires that the individual would otherwise have been in a nursing home because of functional impairment in ADLs. To obtain a waiver to provide services that support IADL functions, in addition to medically related home health services, states have to prove that they would spend no greater amount of Medicaid funds on long-term care (the total for nursing home and HCBS care) than they would in the absence of the proposed waiver.

In many of the states that have HCBS waivers, Medicaid funds for the waiver program are supplemented by state revenues and federal monies obtained through the Older Americans Act and Social Security's (Title 20) block grant social services funds. Most state data on HCBS spending for different types of clients over the same time period are not collected in comparable terms. However, Kane, Kane, and Ladd (1998) estimated expenditures per person age 85 and older, as of 1992, and found that states vary considerably in state and local funds spent on HCBS. Nationwide spending per capita on persons in this age group, was $1,251. Only seven states were above the average. The range was considerable, with New York spending $5,770 per capita, and Mississippi $234 per capita. The average is skewed considerably by New York, which has about 7% of the nation's population of persons age 85 and older (Hobbs, 1996) and spends about 35.8% of the total state and local HCBS dollars in the country.

As is the case with Medicare, the use of Medicaid home health care and expenditures for it have grown dramatically over the years. Between 1975 and 1996 the annual average rate of increase in home health use in Medicaid was 8%, more than 3 times the rate for all types of Medicaid services. During that period, the share of Medicaid expenditures accounted for by home health went from 0.6% to 8.9%, while the share for payments to nursing homes dropped from 35.3% to 24.3%, and the share for hospitals dropped from 27.6% to 20.7%. (The considerable disparity between hospital and home care expenditures will undoubtedly persist because some of the technology used in hospitals cannot be applied in the home.) Since HCBS waivers were authorized in 1981, Medicaid spending on home health services has grown from just $428 million to $10.9 billion, a more than 23-fold increase (Health Care Financing Administration, 1998b).

Public Funding and the Home Care Industry

Paid, formal home care has become a substantial industry as public funding for it has expanded over the past three decades (see chapter 6). By 1996 there were 13,500 home health and hospice agencies in the United States (Haupt, 1998b). Fifty-four percent were proprietary for-profit agencies, 34% were owned by voluntary not-for-profit agencies, and the others were owned by government and other agencies. Eighty-eight percent were Medicare-certified and 86 were Medicaid-certified; eight percent were not certified by either program. Nearly half of the agencies were part of a group or chain of agencies, and 27% were operated by a hospital. In that same year, an estimated 666,000 people were employed by home health care agencies (National Association for Home Care, 1997), including registered nurses; licensed practical nurses; physical, occupational, and speech therapists; home health care aides; social workers, and administrative personnel.

Many long-term care agencies that began as nursing homes are now also providing home care (as well as assisted living and other types of services). Exemplifying this trend is an action taken by the American Association of Homes for the Aging, a trade association for nonprofit nursing homes. In the mid-1990s its name was changed to the American Association of Homes and Services for the Aging.

The total national expenditure for home care providers in 1996, from all sources, was $31.2 billion (Levit et al., 1998). The bulk of it was funded by public sources. Medicare and Medicaid payments totaled $28.4

billion, comprised of Medicare payments totaling $16.8 billion to home health agencies and an estimated $1.6 billion to hospices for home care (see Haupt, 1998a), and $10 billion from Medicaid. About $600 million more was funded by other public sources. Most of the remaining $2.2 billion was primarily paid for out-of-pocket payments by individuals who need home care and their families.

FAMILIES AND HOME CARE

Even with greater availability of public funds for home care services, however, the patient, family, and other informal, unpaid caregivers continue to play a major role in home care.

Caregiving

Although the home care industry has grown tremendously in recent years, families and other "natural" caregivers still provide over 80% of home care on an unpaid basis (see, e.g., Hanley, Alecxih, Wiener, & Kennel, 1990; Norgard & Rodgers, 1997). About 74% of dependent community-based older persons receive all their care from family members or other unpaid sources; approximately 21% receive both formal and informal services, and only about 5% use just formal services (Liu, Manton, & Liu, 1985). The vast majority of family caregivers are women (see Brody, 1990).

The family also plays an important role in obtaining and managing services from paid service providers. When families take the initiative in arranging for paid services, it is usually to supplement their own informal efforts, not to substitute for them. Caregiving by families does not tend to decline significantly when they obtain formal, paid services (Edelman & Hughes, 1990; Tennstedt, Crawford, & McKinlay, 1993).

Even when a substantial amount of paid home care is prescribed by a physician, the family still has major caregiving responsibilities. Periodic home health nursing and visits from physical and occupational therapists and medical social workers, as important as they are, cannot ensure that prescriptions for medications, exercises, and other procedures are complied with properly on an ongoing basis. Contemporary home care often requires that informal and formal care be coordinated effectively to maintain effective, high-quality care (see chapter 4). Moreover, as the expansion of formal home care services has broadened the pool of paid providers, the training and experience of such personnel have become uneven. Patients and families are continually challenged to ensure that formal services are qualitatively adequate.

The need for coordination of informal and formal care has been heightened by the extraordinary advances in medical technologies that can be applied in the home. Ventilator assistance, gastric feeding, intravenous therapy, cardiac monitoring, and other high-tech forms of medical care are now used in home care settings and will proliferate in the future. Their use poses challenges to family caregivers. Families and other caregivers that have 24-hour responsibility for care cannot be wholly dependent on the intermittent and episodic visits of health care professionals.

> Although most recipients of high-tech home care benefit from the periodic assistance of visiting nurses or home hospice workers, much of the time this high-tech is dispensed not by physicians or other specially trained professionals but by patients themselves when capable, or by parents, spouses, adult children, and partners—that is, by ordinary people with no specialized medical training. (Arras, 1995, p. xiii)

Informal caregivers not only need substantial training to use such high-tech applications safely and effectively, but also must implement such training conscientiously.

Paying for Home Care

For those persons not eligible for government-funded benefits, the financial costs of paid home care are substantial. Paying the costs of long-term care out-of-pocket (for a nursing home or home care) can be a catastrophic financial experience for patients and their families.

The Costs

The average annual cost of a year's care in a nursing home was more than $50,700 in 1997 (Health Care Financing Administration, 1998b), a sharp increase from the $37,000 average cost in 1993 (Wiener & Illston, 1996). Although the use of a limited number of services in a home or other community-based setting is less expensive, noninstitutional care for patients who would otherwise be appropriately placed in a nursing home is not cheaper and is often more expensive (Weissert, 1990).

Consider, for example, the findings of a study conducted in nine states on the costs of care for persons with Alzheimer's disease in 1996, who had a combination of both formal and informal care (Leon, Cheng, & Neumann, 1998). Formal, paid home care services—averaged among patients with mild, moderate, and severe dementia—were $8,196 per year. Informal, unpaid care for these patients, often provided when income from employment was sacrificed by the caregiver, was valued at $10,392 by imputing the costs of equivalent services from paid home care workers. Thus, the total annual cost of home care, if paid for out-of-pocket, would have been $18,588. Nursing home care for patients in this study averaged $42,336 that year, or $23,748 more than home care. However, in home care, a variety of expenses in addition to caregiving must be added to the bill in order to get a comparable picture. Among such expenses are lodging, food, utilities, furniture, and a variety of other goods and services that are provided within a nursing home free of charge. Most, if not all, of the "savings" yielded from home care for these patients, $1,979 per month, would be consumed in paying for these expenses. For instance, the U.S. Department of Agriculture, in setting poverty and "near poor" thresholds, assumes that one third of a budget is spent on food. Following this guideline, the home care patient would have a daily food budget of only $21.74 a day.

For the majority of those individuals and families not aided by Medicare, Medicaid, or other government programs, paid home care services are simply unaffordable. In one study about 75% of the informal, unpaid caregivers of dementia patients reported that they did not use paid services because they were unable to pay for them (Eckert & Smyth, 1988).

The cost of care will undoubtedly grow in the future. Price increases in home care have consistently exceeded the general rate of inflation. Trends in labor costs for home care service providers indicate that this pattern will continue (Feldman, 1997).

Private Insurance

Private insurance policies that cover long-term care (including home care) are very expensive for the majority of potential customers. Moreover, benefits are limited with respect to when they first become available and how long they will be paid. A typical good-quality policy will provide benefits of $50 a day for home health care. The benefits are limited, however, with respect to when they first become available and how long they will be paid. From the time that eligibility for benefits is determined there is usually a 90-day waiting period before benefits are paid; in effect, this is a deductible amounting to $4,500 for home care. There is also the problem of price inflation over time. Policies do offer inflation protection for an additional premium, typically at a compounded rate of 5% for benefits. But this additional premium, which varies according to the purchaser's age, is very substantial. For example, for an individual who purchases an insurance policy at the age of 40, the average annual inflation protection fee is 138% of the basic premium; for a purchaser age 65, the average fee is 87% of the premium (Kahn, 1999). Moreover, this additional coverage may not be enough to cover the full rate of inflation in home care costs.

Only about 5% of older persons have any private long-term care insurance (Wiener & Stevenson, 1999) and only 1.1% of home care costs are paid by private insurance (U.S. House of Representatives, 1998). A number of analyses have suggested that even when the product becomes more refined, no more than 20% of older Americans will be able to afford it (Crown, Capitman, & Leutz, 1992; Friedland, 1990; Rivlin & Wiener, 1988; Wiener, Illston, & Hanley, 1994).

A variation on the insurance policy approach to financing long-term care is continuing care retirement communities (CCRCs), which often promise comprehensive health care services, including long-term care, to all members (Sherwood, Ruchlin, Sherwood, & Morris, 1997). According to a report issued by the U.S. General Accounting Office (1997), there are about 350,000 residents living in CCRCs. Only about one third of these, however, provide long-term care for their residents under lifetime contracts in which the CCRC assumes a resident's financial risks for long-term care services. Residents tend to be middle-and upper-income persons who are relatively healthy when they join the community; they pay a substantial entrance fee and monthly charge in return for a promise of "care for life." Because most older people prefer to remain in their own homes rather than to join age-segregated communities, an alternative product termed "life care at home" (LCAH) was developed in the late 1980s and marketed to middle-income customers with lower entry and monthly fees than those of CCRCs (Callahan & Somers, 1994). There are, however, only about 500 LCAH policies in effect (Williams & Temkin-Greener, 1996).

Medicaid "Estate Planning"

Home care patients often use their assets to pay for their care (even including some who have part of their expenses covered by Medicare and Medicaid). In doing so, many "spend down" and eventually deplete their assets to the point that they become poor enough to qualify for Medicaid.

An unknown number of individuals, however, finance home and nursing home long-term care through Medicaid, by legally sheltering their assets and thereby becoming eligible for the program. A burgeoning industry of specialists, so-called Medicaid estate planning attorneys, has provided them with assistance. Because sheltered assets are not counted in Medicaid eligibility determinations, such persons are able to take advantage of a program for the poor, without being poor. Asset sheltering has become a source of considerable concern to the federal and state governments as Medicaid expenditures on long-term care have grown (see Walker & Burwell, 1998).

The frequency of asset sheltering and the sums involved are, in the nature of the case, difficult to ascertain. A few studies have attempted to explore the nature and extent of the phenomenon in selected states (Burwell, 1993; Burwell & Crown, 1995; Walker & Gruman, 1996; Walker, Gruman, & Robison, 1999), but direct documentation is not possible. Through the 1980s and 1990s, Congress enacted laws that made it more difficult to shelter assets and become eligible for Medicaid. Undaunted, however, specialists in Medicaid estate planning have continued to find viable loopholes in the law.

Public/Private Insurance Partnerships

In the early 1990s, The Robert Wood Johnson Foundation financed an experimental program in selected states, in which the prime goal is to reduce Medicaid spending by providing an asset protection incentive for people to purchase long-term care insurance. It is designed to enable middle-class persons to avoid spending down and yet have Medicaid pay for some of their long-term care. At the same time, it seeks to reduce the period that Medicaid will pay for long-term care services that will be needed by an individual. Through this Partnership for Long-Term Care Program, state governments agree to exempt individuals who apply for Medicaid eligibility from having to spend down assets if they have previously had some long-term care paid for by a state-certified private insurance policy.

However, by the end of the 1990s, the sales of these partnership policies had been slow. The partnership programs in New York and California, combined, had yielded sales of only 17,000 policies (Wiener & Stevenson, 1999), even though the two states have 6.1 million persons age 65 and older (Hobbs, 1996). (For fuller discussions of these experiments, see Meiners, 1998; Wiener, 1998.)

ISSUES AND CHALLENGES

Even as the landscape of home care has changed in recent decades, substantial additional changes and challenges lie ahead for patients, families, health professions, and society as we begin the 21st century. A number of major societal dynamics indicate that the need for home care in the years immediately ahead will grow tremendously, even as its provision—*with appropriate quality*—may become increasingly problematic.

Future Growth of the Population Needing Home Care

It is clear that the overall demand for home care will increase substantially in the early decades of the 21st century. When all members of the baby boom—a large birth cohort of 76 million Americans born between 1946 and 1964—reaches the ranks of old age in 2030, the absolute number of people age 65 and older will have doubled from 35 million in the year 2000 to 70 million, and older people will be 20% of the U.S. population. Moreover, the number of persons in advanced old-age ranges will also more than double. The population age 75 and older will have grown from 16.7 million in 2000 to 32.2 million in 2030, and those age 85 and older will have more than doubled, from 4.3 million to 8.6 million (Hobbs, 1996). Rates of disability increase markedly at these advanced old ages. For instance, it is estimated that 6% of people between the ages of 65 and 74 have Alzheimer's disease, but, among persons age 85 and older, as many as 50% show signs of it (National Academy on Aging, 1994). Overall, disability rates among older persons who reside in the community and need home care increase substantially in the older old-age categories, from nearly 23% of those age 65 to 74 who experience difficulty with ADLs to 45% of those age 85 and older (Cassel, Rudberg, & Olshansky, 1992).

Whether rates of disability in old age will increase or decline in the future, however, is a matter on which experts disagree, depending on their assumptions and measures (e.g., Fries, 1989; Manton, Corder, & Stallard, 1993, 1997; Schneider & Guralnik, 1990; Verbrugge, 1989). Yet even those researchers who report a decline in the prevalence of disability at older ages in recent years have emphasized that there will be large absolute increases in the number of older Americans needing long-term care in the decades ahead (e.g., Manton et al., 1993).

This potential future demand for home care services for older people is reflected in estimates of likely expenditures for long-term care in the future. The Congressional Budget Office has projected that total national expenditures (in inflation-adjusted dollars) for services in the home will grow from $37.2 billion in 2000 to $103.3 billion in 2030, an increase of 178% (Congressional Budget Office, 1999).

Predicting whether long-term care needs among people under age 65 will increase or decline is more difficult. One of the principal reasons is that reliable databases for making projections are limited as compared with well-developed national and longitudinal sources available regarding the older population (LaPlante, 1993). Moreover, the numbers involved with respect to various disabling conditions—such as spinal cord injury, cerebral palsy, and mental retardation—are relatively small and much more susceptible to changing conditions.

Yet experts agree that the number of younger disabled persons has grown in recent years, and this trend may well persist (Ross, 1994). New technologies and increased access to medical care continue to enable more people to survive injuries and other conditions that were heretofore fatal, and thereby live for many years with ADL limitations. For example, 80% to 90% of persons with lupus can now expect a normal life span (Huber, 1997). In addition, biomedical advances have enabled many more children with developmental disabilities and low-birth-weight infants to survive much longer than in the past, and have extended years in which they need long-term care.

Family Caregiving in the Future

Although families presently provide the bulk of home care, the capacities and willingness of family members to provide care may decline during the next few decades. One reason is that the fertility rate for baby boomers has been considerably lower than that of preceding birth cohorts (Stone, 1999). Thus, when baby boomers reach advanced older ages and the need for caregiving will increase, the ratio of potential adult children caregivers to parents needing care will be smaller than it is today.

Another reason is that the family, as a fundamental unit of social organization, has been undergoing profound transformations that will become more fully manifest over the next few decades as baby boomers reach old age. The striking growth of single-parent households, the growing participation of women in the labor force, the high incidence of divorce and remarriage (differentially higher for men), all entail complicated changes in the structure of household and kinship roles and relationships. There will be an increasing number of "blended families," reflecting multiple lines of descent through multiple marriages and the birth of children outside wedlock through other partners. This growth in the incidence of step-and half-relatives will make for a dramatic new turn in family structure in the coming decades. Already, such blended families constitute about half of all households with children (National Academy on Aging, 1994). One possible implication of these changes is that kinship networks in the near future will become more complex, attenuated, and diffuse (Bengtson, Rosenthal, & Burton, 1990). If changes in the intensity of kinship relations significantly erode the capacity and sense of obligation to provide informal care, demands for governmental support to pay for home health services may increase accordingly.

Challenges in Information Technology

In situations when family and paid caregivers are unavailable at any given time, advances in information and computer technology have made home care more viable than in the past (see chapter 3). For example, personal emergency response systems have enabled many vulnerable patients to feel more secure when they are home alone.

Yet many more developments in this area are on the drawing boards and can be developed in the future. At the very least, as Coughlin (1999) noted, "Systems that make full use of existing communications infrastructure can be used to ensure that medicine has been taken, that heart or other physical functions are well, and that minor symptoms are not indicators of a large problem—problems that if left untreated might result in hospitalization for the individual and higher healthcare costs for society" (p. 4). Indeed, according to Sheridan and Thompson (1999), development of such systems is currently under way.

> There are many current efforts to design, test, and market new devices to be used in the home or nursing facility, either by patients themselves or by trained health care workers. These devices are often smaller and more user-friendly versions of standard in-hospital devices that measure such things as temperature, pulse rate, blood pressure, and blood oxygen saturation. Such devices are also getting smarter, and computer chips integral to the devices indicate whether the readings are in normal range, are abnormal, or are somewhere in between. New prototypes of some such devices are getting so small and nonintrusive as to be wearable as finger rings, [B]and-aids, or articles of jewelry or clothing. Such devices have the prospect of providing round-the-clock continuous monitoring of important physiological variables. (pp. 7–8)

Many similar sophisticated devices are also possible. Sheridan and Thompson offer a vision of home care use of a heart-monitoring apparatus that periodically connects automatically to a computer in a local hospital and downloads stored data. This enables an electronic record of the patient's status to be updated in the hospital computer.

The frontiers of technological development in the service of home care patients offer a wide range of possibilities. Robotic devices can assist in mobility and control. It is well within the range of current technology to create "smart houses," residential environments that can actively respond to, accommodate to, and compensate for physical and cognitive functional deficits. Smart houses can be integrated with larger networks of health care professionals and other service providers, as well as families and friends. In effect, virtual "smart communities" can be developed, defined by the flow of information and largely independent of physical proximity. These and other potential developments are essentially a matter of systems engineering. As the aging of the baby boom brings new visibility to the market for meeting home care needs, researchers and entrepreneurs will likely find creative ways to integrate and apply technologies to meet the needs of home care patients.

Challenges to the Health Care Professions

Health care professions will be challenged to become more effectively oriented toward home care in the years ahead. Physicians have a key role to play in home care. They are responsible for defining the need for home care and must certify specific needs for formal services provided by home care agencies and health professionals if those services are to be eligible for reimbursement by Medicare and Medicaid. Yet the medical profession has given too little attention to health care services for patients at home. Physicians have little experience with the settings, circumstances, or conditions under which home care can or will be provided. Home care agencies and nurses decry the lack of physician involvement. Too many physicians do little to oversee or monitor home care they prescribe and work at a distance from those providing home care. In 1995, to encourage greater physician involvement in overseeing and ensuring the quality of home care, HCFA began paying physicians at the rate of $81 per patient for oversight of home care requiring at least 30 minutes. Yet, even with this financial incentive, physicians have scant involvement in home care.

Medical education gives little, if any, attention to training physicians with respect to issues involved in home care, even though the technology prescribed for use in the home, under supervision of patient, family, friends, and health professionals, often requires physician involvement. As the demand for home care continues to grow, the medical education establishment will be challenged to do a much better job of orienting physicians to the complexities of home care and the importance of their involvement in it.

Similarly, nursing and physical therapy are keys to home health care. Yet education in these professions has paid too little attention to their growing role in home care. Fortunately, this is being corrected, but the need for nurses and other health care professionals trained in home care is growing rapidly. Concomitantly, as more and more hospital beds close, education and training programs in home care will become ever more important to these professions.

An important aspect of challenges to health professionals, and health care administrators as well, is to work toward making home health care part of an integrated, seamless system of health care. Too frequently home care is neither viewed nor functions as part of a continuum of health care, including care in hospitals, physicians' offices, clinics, rehabilitation or social services, and ambulatory medical and surgical services. As is often the case with other segments of medical care, home care is treated as if it were separate and autonomous. Increased recognition of home care as part of a continuum of health care will improve its quality, as well as the overall quality of health care systems. Effective implementation of this vision may enable policymakers, in turn, to recognize that adequate funding of home health services is as important to the health of Americans as funding care in hospitals and other settings.

The Challenge to Public Policy

Perhaps the greatest challenge that lies ahead in the arena of home health care is a societal one—adequate public financing to meet the vastly increased demand for formal services that will develop in the decades ahead, while ensuring that the services provided are of appropriate quality (see chapter 10). As noted above, under current law public spending for home care is projected to nearly triple by 2030.

The Ups and Downs of the Early 1990s

From the late 1980s through the early 1990s, the prospects for expanded government financing of home health services seemed good. A number of national policymakers were sympathetic to the dilemmas confronting middle-income individuals who needed long-term care—their inability to pay out-of-pocket for services or for private insurance that provides adequate coverage, and the anxieties of spending down their modest assets in the process of becoming eligible for Medicaid. In the early 1990s advocates for the elderly and younger disabled persons were optimistic that the federal government would establish a new program for funding long-term care that would not be means-tested, as is Medicaid.

A number of legislative bills introduced from 1989 to 1994 included some version of such a program, including President Clinton's failed proposal for health care reform (see Binstock, 1994). None of these proposals became law. The major reason was that in the context of "balanced budget" politics any substantial version of such a program would cost tens of billions of dollars each year just at the outset.

By the mid-1990s, optimism regarding expanded governmental funding for long-term care was quashed. A new Republican majority in the 104th Congress reversed the focus on long-term care from expansion to retraction. It proposed to limit federal spending on Medicaid and Medicare, as part of a broader agenda for balancing the annual federal budget and redistributing responsibilities of the federal government to the states (see Binstock, 1997).

Policy Agenda for the Private Insurance Industry

Following the disappearance from the national policy agenda of any attempts to establish new or expanded programs of governmental funding for long-term care, Congress began to promote the growth of private long-term care insurance. Partial tax credits and deductibility for premiums paid for insurance policies were established. At the same time (as discussed above), Congress attempted to make things difficult for the long-term care insurance industry's chief competitors in the private market—Medicaid estate planners—by closing loopholes through which assets could be sheltered.

During the 1990s the volume of long-term care insurance business increased fourfold, with aggregate annual premiums paid growing from $302 million to $1.2 billion (Miller, Andrews, & Cohen, 1999). The Congressional Budget Office (1999) foresees continued growth in the industry's coverage of home care expenses, projecting that 10.6% of home care costs for older persons will be financed by private insurance in 2020.

The industry itself is optimistic that its market will grow substantially in the years ahead, as its products and marketing strategies continue to improve and the baby boom cohort grows old. Moreover, it has established an agenda of public policy priorities through which it hopes to promote its growth (Kahn, 1999). The industry seeks 100% deductibility for long-term care insurance premiums, a goal reflected in House Resolution 1261, a bipartisan bill cosponsored by 15 members of the U.S. House of Representatives in 1999. It is also working to establish tax incentives at the state level, as well as federal laws to permit the use of pretax dollars to purchase long-term care insurance through employee flexible spending accounts, individual retirement accounts, and 401(k)s. Not surprisingly, public policy analysts who are not part of the insurance industry have suggested that the tax dollars spent on subsidizing private insurance might alternatively be spent on funding long-term care through the public sector (e.g., Feder, 1999).

Retrenchment in Public Spending

With the passage of the Balanced Budget Act of 1997 (BBA97), the dominant policy trend with respect to home care became efforts to limiting government expenditures. Changes in reimbursement for home health care, pursuant to BBA97, were intended to curtail growth in the home care industry, increase efficiency, reduce fraud, and achieve an estimated $16.2 billion in savings over 5 years. Pre-BBA97 projections had estimated a 9.5% annual growth for this period (Komisar & Feder, 1998).

Following BBA97, the rapid growth of the home care industry has been reversed. Prior to the adoption of a prospective payment system for Medicare home health care (scheduled for late 1999, but now postponed for implementation until 2001), an interim payment system was established. The result is that reimbursements to home health agencies are now averaging 31% less than they were before BBA97, and more than a tenth of the nation's Medicare-certified home health agencies have been closed (Flaherty, 1998). Many patients who need professional home care services are not getting them. Moreover, for those who are getting services, issues have arisen regarding quality of care because home health care visits are fewer and shorter under the new policies. (The actual relationship between cost and quality in home care, or what economists would term "the cost-of-quality curve," is not truly known; see Binstock & Spector, 1997).

Managed Care and Home Care

The spread of managed care, in both the Medicare and Medicaid programs, has also raised issues concerning the quality of home care. Under managed care, home health agencies operate under fixed budgets. To stay within these budgets, they have changed their staffing patterns, the number of home visits that are made, and the length of visits (see chapter 7 for a discussion of how these and other variables affect resource consumption).

Studies have indicated that health status outcomes for patients who receive home care under managed care arrangements are worse than for those who receive it under the traditional fee-for-service system (see chapter 8). Yet experimental demonstration efforts suggest that managed care outcomes need not be worse if home care is actively planned and supervised by a hospital-based team of health professionals, including physicians (see chapter 9).

President Clinton's 1999 Initiative

Federal expansion of benefits for home care was placed back on the policy agenda in 1999 when President Clinton announced a "Long-term

Care Initiative" (see White House, 1999a, 1999b, 1999c). His proposal included an annual $1,000 nonrefundable tax credit for a family caregiver who houses and cares for severely disabled individuals—those with three or more ADL limitations or "comparable cognitive impairment"— regardless of whether they purchase formal services. The tax credit would begin to phase out for couples with $110,000 in income (eliminated entirely at $130,000), and for unmarried taxpayers at $75,000 (eliminated at $95,000). In the absence of family caregiving, impaired individuals would also be eligible for the tax credit, whether they are residing at home or in institutions. Receipt of the tax credit would not require itemization of bills for caregiving, but simply a certification by a physician that the patient's condition meets the eligibility requirements concerning impairments in ADLs or cognition. The Clinton administration estimated that this program would cost $5.5 billion over 5 years, and that three fourths of the credits would go to relatives of people needing home care.

The proposed nonrefundable tax credit, of course, would be of little use to relatively low-income persons who have little or no income tax liability. As Joshua Wiener, an expert in long-term care policy, commented, "You have to pay some taxes to qualify, and 40% of the elderly pay no income taxes at all, primarily because substantial amounts of Social Security are not counted as income for tax purposes" (Pear, 1999). Moreover, as indicated earlier in this chapter, $1,000 is a negligible sum when placed within the total context of the costs of long-term care for individuals and families.

Nonetheless, Clinton's proposal was the first to address the needs of family caregivers. In addition to the tax credit, it also called for the establishment of a meagerly funded National Caregiver Support Program ($625 million over 5 years). The program would have states create "one-stop shops" that provide quality respite care and other support services; critical information about community-based long-term care services; counseling and support programs for caregivers to help them cope with their responsibilities; and training for family members in the use of high-technology home care interventions, such as feeding tubes. Also included was a $10 million program to educate Medicare enrollees with respect to long-care services and public funding for them. In addition, Clinton's initiative called for $110 million over 5 years to expand the Medicaid HCBS program, and an additional $110 million to encourage use of HCBS in federally financed housing projects for the elderly. Finally, the administration proposed that the federal government become a "model employer" by offering private long-term care insurance as an employee benefit to federal personnel, at an estimated cost to the government of $15 million over 5 years.

Although, President Clinton's initiative was extremely modest in terms of funding and scope, it had substantial symbolic importance. Expansion of public funding for long-term care had vanished from the national policy agenda following the failure of his health care reform proposal in 1994. But in 1999, a year when the issues of reforming Social Security and Medicare had high visibility, the president revived public attention to the notion that the federal government has a greater role to play in long-term care funding, especially in the area of home care.

Future Prospects

The appropriate balance of public and private responsibility for financing long-term care will be a major societal issue in the years immediately ahead (see Walker, Bradley, & Wetle, 1998). Out-of-pocket payments for care are becoming larger and increasingly unaffordable for many; neither the projected income and asset status of members of the baby boom cohort nor the dynamics of the market (at this time) indicate that these trends will abate. Only a minority of older persons may be able to afford premiums for private long-term care insurance. Broad societal trends suggest that informal, unpaid care by family members may become less feasible in the future than it is today.

When baby boomers reach old age, many of them and their families may look to government to subsidize their long-term care, in general, and home care, in particular. Yet even the assistance that government programs now provide through Medicare and Medicaid is seriously threatened by contemporary federal and state budgetary politics. In the present political context public resources for home care are likely to be even less available, in relation to the need for care, than they have been to date. As the demand for long-term care increases in the decades ahead, what is likely to happen?

Perhaps the entrance of the baby boom into the ranks of old age may precipitate a grassroots movement that will revitalize political awareness of the problem of long-term care financing as a major issue in American society. Such a movement might well be joined by millions of younger disabled persons and their advocates, although the constituencies of the elderly and the disabled have a checkered history of working as allies because of differing philosophical and political concerns (see Binstock, 1992, 1994).

The prospects of success for such a grassroots movement will probably depend on effective promulgation of the notion that long-term care, including home care, is an essential part of *health care* (a notion that traditionally has been anathema to the younger disabled constituency). This would make it possible for long-term care to receive adequate attention in more general policy debates about the future of American health care.

For most of the 20th century, care at home and in nursing homes has been eclipsed by the glamour and prestige of hospital-based medical care that is inherently dramatic because it deals with acute episodes of illnesses and trauma, and the relatively "high-tech" and "quick-fix" dimensions of diagnosis and intervention that have been associated with them. Long-term care has not even been covered through traditional health insurance mechanisms such as employee benefit plans. When concerns are expressed about the fact that 43 million Americans are not covered by health insurance, coverage for long-term care is not part of the discussion.

It is possible that home care will come to be perceived more widely as part of the continuum of health care that is needed by all of us. As the aging of the baby boom cohort engenders a formidable volume of need for care, the importance of long-term care—including the difficulties of financing it, and the challenges of delivering it effectively—is likely to become increasingly accepted throughout American society. Such acceptance could bring with it a widespread understanding that long-term care is health care by another name. This perception may enfold long-term care into a shared understanding of justice in health care in which ensuring access to home care is as much of a public responsibility as ensuring access to other kinds of health care. If so, the political context may be more favorable for even a substantially greater public role in financing long-term care than there is today. In the meantime, it will be essential for methods to be developed that will enable individuals, families, and communities to address their needs for home care more effectively, even without expanded public funding.

REFERENCES

Arras, J. D. (Ed.). (1995). *Bringing the hospital home: Ethical and social implications of high-tech home care.* Baltimore, MD: Johns Hopkins University Press.

Bengtson, V. L., Rosenthal, C., & Burton, L. (1990). Families and aging: Diversity and heterogeneity. In R. H. Binstock & L. K. George (Eds.), *Handbook of aging and the social sciences* (3rd ed., pp. 263–287). San Diego, CA: Academic Press.

Benjamin, A. E. (1993). An historical perspective on home care policy. *Milbank Quarterly, 71,* 129–166.

Binstock, R. H. (1992). Aging, disability, and long-term care: The politics of common ground. *Generations, 16*(2), 83–88.

———. (1994). Older Americans and health care reform in the 1990s. In P. V. Rosenau (Ed.), *Health Care Reform in the Nineties* (pp. 213–235). Thousand Oaks, CA: Sage Publications.

———. (1997). The old-age lobby in a new political era. In R. B. Hudson (Ed.), *The future of age-based policy* (pp. 56–74). Baltimore, MD: Johns Hopkins University Press.

Binstock, R. H., & Spector, W. D. (1997). Five priority areas for research on long-term care. *Health Services Research, 32,* 715–730.

Bishop, C., & Skwara, K. C. (1993). Recent growth of Medicare home health. *Health Affairs, 12*(3), 95–110.

Brody, E. (1990). *Women in the middle: Their parent-care years.* New York: Springer Publishing.

Burwell, B. (1993). *State responses to Medicaid estate planning.* Cambridge, MA: SysteMetrics.

Burwell, B., & Crown, W. H. (1995). *Medicaid estate planning in the aftermath of OBRA '93.* Cambridge, MA: The MEDSTAT Group.

Callahan, J. J., Jr., & Somers., S. A. (1994). Life care at home: The experience and the issues. *Compensation and Benefits Management, 10*(2), 49–60.

Callender, M., & LaVor, J. (1975). *Home health care development: Problems, and potential.* Washington, DC: U.S. Department of Health, Education, and Welfare.

Cassel, C. K., Rudberg, M. A., & Olshansky, S. J. (1992). The price of success: Health care in an aging society. *Health Affairs, 11*(2), 87–99.

Cole, T. R. (1996). The evolution of long-term care in America. In R. H. Binstock, L. E. Cluff, & O. von Mering (Eds.), *The future of long-term care: Social and policy issues* (pp. 19–47). Baltimore, MD: Johns Hopkins University Press.

Congressional Budget Office. (1999). Projections of expenditures for long-term care services for the elderly. Washington, DC: U.S. Government Printing Office.

Coughlin, J. F. (1999). Setting a national policy agenda for technology and health aging. *Public Policy and Aging Report, 10*(1), 1, 3–6.

Crown, W. H., Capitman, J., & Leutz, W. N. (1992). Economic rationality, the affordability of private long-term care insurance, and the role for public policy. *Gerontologist, 32,* 478–485.

Eckert, S. K., & Smyth, K. (1988). *A case study of methods of locating and arranging health and long-term care for persons with dementia.* Washington, DC: Office of Technology Assessment, Congress of the United States.

Edelman, P., & Hughes, S. (1990). The impact of community care on provision of informal care to homebound elderly persons. *Journals of Gerontology: Social Sciences, 45,* S874–S884.

Feder, J. (1999, April). *The policy context for the long-term care debate.* Paper presented at the conference "Financing Long-Term Care: Policy Options and Their Economic Impact," sponsored by the Council on the Economic Impact of Health System Change, Brandeis University, Waltham, MA.

Feldman, P. H. (1997). Labor market issues in home care. In D. F. Fox & C. Raphael (Eds.), *Home-based care for a new century* (pp. 155–183). Malden, MA: Blackwell Publishers.

Flaherty, M. (1998). Close to closure: Home care feels the squeeze. *Aging Today, 19*(6), 1, 6.

Friedland, R. (1990). *Facing the costs of long-term care: An EBRI-ERF policy study.* Washington, DC: Employee Benefits Research Institute.

Fries, J. F. (1989). The compression of morbidity: Near or far? *Milbank Quarterly, 67,* 208–232.

Hanley, R. J., Alecxih, L. M. B., Wiener, J. M., & Kennel, D. L. (1990). Predicting elderly nursing home admissions: Results from the 1982–86 National Long-Term Care Survey. *Research on Aging, 12,* 199–228.

Haupt, B. J. (1998a). *Characteristics of hospice care users: 1996 National Home and Hospice Care Survey* (Advance Data from Vital and Health Statistics of the Centers for Disease Control and Prevention, No. 299). Hyattsville, MD: National Center for Health Statistics, U.S. Department of Health and Human Services.

_____. (1998b). *An overview of home health and hospice care patients: 1996 National Home and Hospice Care Survey* (Advance Data from Vital and Health Statistics of the Centers for Disease Control and Prevention, No. 297). Hyattsville, MD: National Center for Health Statistics, U.S. Department of Health and Human Services.

Health Care Financing Administration. (1998a). Medicare and Medicaid statistical supplement, 1998. *Health Care Financing Review.*

_____. (1998b). Information provided by Helen Lazenby of the Office of National Cost Estimates.

Hobbs, F. B. (1996). *65+ in the United States* (U.S. Bureau of the Census, Current Population Reports, Special Studies, P23–190). Washington, DC: U.S. Government Printing Office.

Huber, J. (1997). Interview with Huber, executive director of the Lupus Foundation, conducted by Robert Binstock, June 30.

Kahn, C. N., III. (1999, April). *Possibilities of change: Insurer's perspectives.*

Paper presented at the conference "Financing Long-Term Care: Policy Options and Their Economic Impact," sponsored by the Council on the Economic Impact of Health System Change, Brandeis University, Waltham, MA.

Kane, R. A., Kane, R. L., & Ladd, R. C. (1998). *The heart of long-term care.* New York: Oxford University Press.

Kemper, P. R., Brown, R. S., Carcagno, G. J., Applebaum, R. A., Christianson, J. B., Corson, W., Dunstan, S. M., Grannemann, T., Harrigan, M., Holden, N., Phillips, B. R., Schore, J., Thornton, C., Wooldridge, J., & Skidmore, F. (1988). The evaluation of the national long-term care demonstration [Special issue]. *Health Services Research, 23*(1).

Komisar, H., & Feder, J. (1998). *The Balanced Budget Act of 1997: Effects on Medicare's home health benefit and beneficiaries who need long-term care.* New York: The Commonwealth Fund.

LaPlante, M. P. (1993). *Disability statistics report: State estimates of disability in America.* Washington, DC: National Institute on Disability and Rehabilitation Research, U.S. Department of Education, Office of Special Education and Rehabilitative Services.

Leon, J. L., Cheng, C.-K., & Neumann, P. J. (1998). Alzheimer's disease and care: Costs and potential savings. *Health Affairs, 17*(6), 206–216.

Levit, K., Cowan, C., Braden, B., Stiller, J., Sensenig, A., & Lazenby, H. (1998). National health expenditures in 1997: More slow growth. *Health Affairs, 17*(6), 99–110.

Liu, K., Manton, K. M., & Liu, B. M. (1985). Home care expenses for the disabled elderly. *Health Care Financing Review, 7*(2), 51–58.

Manton, K. G., Corder, L. S., & Stallard, E. (1993). Estimates of change in chronic disability and institutional incidence and prevalence rates in the U.S. elderly population from the 1982, 1984, and 1989 National Long Term Care Survey. *Journal of Gerontology: Social Sciences, 48,* S153–S166.

_____. (1997). Chronic disability trends in elderly United States populations: 1982–1994. *Proceedings of the National Academy of Sciences, USA, 94,* 2593–2598.

Meiners, M. R. (1998). Public-private partnerships in long-term care. In L. C. Walker, E. H. Bradley, & T. Wetle (Eds.), *Public and private responsibilities in long-term care: Finding the balance* (pp. 115–133). Baltimore, MD: Johns Hopkins University Press.

Miller, J., Andrews, K., & Cohen, M. A. (1999, April). *The health of the LTC insurance industry in the United States: Looking toward the 21st century.* Paper presented at the conference "Financing Long-Term Care: Policy Options and Their Economic Impact," sponsored by the Council on the Economic Impact of Health System Change, Brandeis University, Waltham, MA.

National Academy on Aging. (1994). *Old age in the 21st century.* Washington, DC: Syracuse University.
National Association for Home Care. (1997). *Basic statistics about home care, 1997.* www.nahc.org/Consumer/hestats.htm.
Norgard, T. M., & Rodgers, W. L. (1997) Patterns of in-home care among elderly black and white Americans [Special issue]. *Journals of Gerontology: Series B, 52B,* 93–101.
Pear, R. (1999, January 4). Clinton seeks aid for care of those with chronic ills. *New York Times,* p. 1.
Rivlin, A. M., & Wiener, J. M. (1988). *Caring for the disabled elderly: Who will pay?* Washington, DC: The Brookings Institution.
Ross, J. L. (1994). *Long-term care: Demography, dollars, and dissatisfaction drive reform* (Testimony before the Special Committee on Aging, U.S. Senate, April 12. U.S. GAO/T-HEHS-94–140). Washington, DC: U.S. Government Printing Office.
Schneider, E. L.,& Guralnik, J. M. (1990). The aging of America: Impact on health care costs. *Journal of the American Medical Association, 263,* 2335–2340.
Sheridan, T. B., & Thompson, J. M. (1999). Today's communications technology—tomorrow's health care. *Public Policy and Aging Report, 10*(1), 7–9.
Sherwood, S., Ruchlin, H. S., Sherwood, C. C., & Morris, S. A. (1997*). Continuing care retirement communities.* Baltimore, MD: Johns Hopkins University Press.
Stone, R. I. (1999, April). *The changing federal role in financing long-term care.* Paper presented at the conference "Financing Long-Term Care: Policy Options and Their Economic Impact," sponsored by the Council on the Economic Impact of Health System Change, Brandeis University, Waltham, MA.
Tennstedt, S. L., Crawford, S. L., & McKinlay, J. B. (1993). Is family care on the decline? A longitudinal investigation of the substitution of formal long-term care services for informal care. *Milbank Quarterly, 71,* 601–624.
U.S. General Accounting Office. (1997). *Health care services: How continuing care retirement communities manage services for the elderly.* Washington, DC: U.S. Government Printing Office.
U.S. House of Representatives, Committee on Ways and Means. (1998). *1998 Green Book.* Washington, DC: U.S. Government Printing Office.
Verbrugge, L. M. (1989). Recent, present, and future health of American adults. In L. Breslow, J. E. Fielding, & L. B. Lave (Eds.), *Annual review of public health* (Vol. 10, pp. 333–361). Palo Alto, CA: Annual Reviews.
Vladeck, B. C. (1980*). Unloving care.* New York: Basic Books.
Walker, L. C., Bradley, E. H., & T. Wetle (Eds). (1998). *Public and private*

responsibilities in long-term care: Finding the balance. Baltimore, MD: Johns Hopkins University Press.

Walker, L. C., & Burwell, B. (1998). Access to public resources: Regulating asset transfers for long-term care. In L. C. Walker, E. H. Bradley, & T. Wetle, eds., *Public and private responsibilities in long-term care: Finding the balance* (pp. 165–180). Baltimore, MD: Johns Hopkins University Press.

Walker, L. C., & Gruman, C. (1996). *Medicaid estate planning for nursing home care in Connecticut: Policies, practices, and perceptions reported by Connecticut Medicaid eligibility workers.* Hartford, CT: Braceland Center for Mental Health and Aging.

Walker, L. C., Gruman, C., & Robison, J. (1999). Medicaid eligibility workers discuss Medicaid estate planning for nursing home care. *Gerontologist, 39,* 201–208.

Weissert, W. G. (1990). Strategies for reducing home-care expenditures. *Generations, 14*(2), 42–44.

White House. (1999a). President Clinton and Vice President Gore unveil historic long-term care initiative to support family caregivers and help address growing long-term care needs. Office of the Press Secretary, January 4. www.pub.whitehouse.gove/uri-res/12R?urn:pdi://poma.eop.gov.us/1999/1/4/3.text.1.

———. (1999b). Remarks by the President on long-term health care initiative. Office of the Press Secretary, January 4. www.pub.whitehouse.gove/uri-res/12R?urn:pdi://poma.eop.gov.us/1999/1/4/6.text.1.

———. (1999c). Press briefing by Secretary of Health and Human Services Donna Shalala, Director of OPM Janice Lachance, Deputy Assistant to the President for Health Care Chris Jennings. January 4. www.pub.whitehouse.gove/uri-res/12R?urn:pdi://poma.eop.gov.us/1999/1/4/7.text.1.

Wiener, J. M. (1998). Jump starting the market: Public subsidies for private long-term care insurance. In L. C. Walker, E. H. Bradley, & T. Wetl (Eds.), *Public and private responsibilities in long-term care: Finding the balance* (pp. 134–149). Baltimore, MD: Johns Hopkins University Press.

Wiener, J. M., & Illston, L. H. (1996). Health care financing and organization for the elderly. In R. H. Binstock & L. K. George (Eds.), *Handbook of aging and the social sciences* (4th ed., pp. 427–445). San Diego, CA: Academic Press.

Wiener, J. M., Illston, L. H., & Hanley, R. J. (1994). *Sharing the burden: Strategies for public and private long-term care insurance.* Washington, DC: The Brookings Institution.

Wiener, J. M., & Stevenson, D. G. (1999, April). *Assessing the new federalism: Long-term care for the elderly and state policy.* Paper presented at the conference "Financing Long-Term Care: Policy Options and Their Economic Impact," sponsored by the Council on the Economic Impact of Health System Change, Brandeis University, Waltham, MA.

Williams, T. F., & Temkin-Greener, H. (1996). Older people, dependency, and trends in supportive care. In R. H. Binstock, L. E. Cluff, & O. von Mering (Eds.), *The future of long-term care: Social and policy issues* (pp. 51–74). Baltimore, MD: Johns Hopkins University Press.

CHAPTER 2

The Changing Health and Social Environments of Home Care

Donna M. Cox
Marcia G. Ory

The end of the 20th century brought unprecedented growth in the numbers of older people as well as in the numbers of those who need help with daily living. From 1960 to 2000 the population of Americans age 65 and older doubled, reaching nearly 35 million persons (U.S. Bureau of the Census, 1997). The oldest-old population, those 85 years and older, is expected to more than quadruple, from 4 million in 2000 to 18 million by 2050 (U.S. Bureau of the Census, 1996). Such population aging has dramatic implications for health care as the elderly are the heaviest consumers of health care services and claim approximately three fifths of the health bill funded by public monies (U.S. Bureau of the Census, 1996).

Questions abound about how health and social care systems will adapt to meet the service demands of an aging and increasingly diverse population. Despite the maturing of the long-term care (LTC) system over the past 25 years, issues of need, use, and outcome are still paramount.

States, which have long been burdened by the costs of LTC, have introduced innovative strategies to reduce unnecessary and costly institutional placements (American Association of Homes and Services for the Aging, 1997; Saucier & Riley, 1994; Snow, 1995). They continue to search for ways to improve access to LTC services, as well as quality and coordination of care. LTC services provided in the home, whether one's own home or that of another, will become of even greater importance as public and private entities respond to demographic, market, and policy pressures.

The purpose of this chapter is to examine home care in the context of the rapidly changing health and social environments at the turn of the 21st century. It begins with a brief overview of the population needing long-term care. It then focuses on the home care industry that serves a large segment of this population, with attention to changes in the industry and current trends in the use of home care. Next, it delineates how home care has evolved to its present-day forms, with new models and considerable expansion in the concept of home care. Finally, it sets forth a continuing research agenda for the field of home care.

WHO NEEDS LONG-TERM CARE?

Long-term care refers to a range of personal, social, and medical services provided to people of all ages who need some level of personal care with major life activities (Rabin & Stockton, 1987). The services needed may vary depending on the individual's coping skills, disabilities, or impairments resulting from chronic illness, injury, or other conditions (Bringewatt, 1995). While LTC services most often address personal and social needs of the disabled (e.g., eating, toileting, ambulating, shopping), medical care requiring use of advanced technology and skill in the home is becoming more common.

Chronic Illnesses and Comorbidities

Although the majority of older people remain relatively healthy and functional until the eighth decade, there is an increased likelihood that they will have one or more chronic illnesses leading to disability and dependency. Comorbidities are common. Over 70% of women and 50% of men report having two or more of nine common conditions—arthritis, hypertension, cataracts, heart disease, varicose veins, diabetes, cancer, osteoporosis or hip fracture, and stroke (U.S. Bureau of the Census, 1996). Stroke, chronic obstructive pulmonary disease, and heart failure are the three diagnosis-related groupings that are most likely to contribute to increases in home LTC needs (Dey, 1996).

Increased LTC Needs With Aging

Thus, Americans who live beyond the age of 65 can anticipate a growing likelihood of needing assistance in performing personal care and home management tasks. Problems in activities of daily living (ADLs) trigger the need for long-term care and benefits are often based on having two or more problems in ADLs (Kassner & Bectel, 1998). Among the civilian noninstitutionalized population, only 1% of persons 50 to 64 reported needing assistance in two or more ADLs, as compared to 2% of those age 65 to 74 years, 5% of those age 75 to 84 years, and 11% of those age 85 and older (Kassner & Bechtel, 1998). Approximately half of the civilian non-institutionalized oldest-old population has at least one functional disability (Cohen & Van Nostrand, 1995; U.S. Bureau of the Census, 1996).

Health Improvements

Recent findings indicating a decline in the rate of disability for older persons during the 1980s suggest that today's elderly may be healthier than earlier generations (Manton, Stallard, & Corder, 1995). Improvements in education, nutrition, preventive health care, and the adoption of healthier lifestyles are among the reasons cited for the reported decline. However, the extent to which disability rates will continue to fall is unknown. Regardless, population aging will result in an overall increase in the burden of disability, and subgroups within the older population are not experiencing the same gains as Whites and those of higher education (Manton, Corder, & Stallard, 1997; Waidmann & Manton, 1998).

Long-term Care Across the Life Span

The LTC population is commonly assumed to consist only of elderly people who have become frail and dependent. This is a misperception. Obtaining and paying for LTC are not strictly issues for the elderly.

While the majority of persons in need of LTC are 65 or older, over 40% of those with long-term care needs are children or working-age adults (Stone, 1995). These age differences create distinct challenges for LTC systems. Even though the nonaged and aged receiving LTC may have similar personal care needs, there are important differences between them that relate to personal aspirations and values. These differences influence what services are required and how they will be provided (Stone, 1995). Moreover, children and nonaged adults lack private insurance coverage or are underinsured. They are more likely to rely on Medicaid or some other state program for assistance. In comparison, those eligible for Medicare, primarily persons age 65 years or older, may receive limited coverage for home care services and skilled nursing facility care. In addition, 13% of this population are also eligible for Medicaid coverage, which covers institutional LTC and, in some states, home care and personal care services.

THE CHANGING HOME CARE INDUSTRY

For most older persons, remaining in one's home or the home of another is preferred over nursing home placement. The constant growth in Medicaid program spending and the increasing demand for services have prompted states to undertake change in state long-term care systems. To reduce reliance on institutional settings, states have adopted policies to control the supply of nursing facility beds, while experimenting with programs and waivers to promote the development of home and community-based services. Some states (e.g., Oregon) have invested heavily to decrease reliance on institutional settings for long-term care (Kane, Kane, & Ladd, 1998). Even in the face of limited funding, the demand for alternative living arrangements, such as assisted living, and in-home and community-based services, will remain strong. The force of this demand is notably reflected in the home care sector, the fastest growing segment of long-term care.

Definitions of Home Care

Traditional images of home care consist of visiting nurses performing dressing changes and doing blood pressures. This is a very limited perception. *Home care* refers to a broad array of professional and paraprofessional postacute and long-term medical and social services provided in nonmedical residential settings. Providers range from the physician, nurse, and various types of therapists on one end of the continuum, to housekeeping, chore, and volunteer services at the other (Benjamin, 1993). Within a changing environment that seeks greater flexibility in meeting the demands of those needing long-term care, *home* is also broadly defined. In this case, *home* refers to any residential setting in which formal medical services are not provided as part of the housing component, although supportive services may be. Residential settings may be a detached home, an apartment in a family member's home or large complex, an assisted living facility, or a unit in a congregate housing arrangement with supportive services. Although these settings may include board and care arrangements, they do not include nursing homes or, generally speaking, day care outside the home (Ory & Duncker, 1992).

Home Care Industry and Services

The home care industry (see chapter 6) is as dynamic and as diverse as the population it serves. Home care services may be provided by home health care agencies, home care aide organizations, or hospices. They may be certified or noncertified, freestanding agencies or hospital-based. Most home health care agencies and hospices are Medicare-certified (National Association for Home Care, 1998). In 1967 freestanding, public health agencies dominated the industry; hospital-based and proprietary agencies together represented only about one quarter of all agencies. Today, proprietary agencies outnumber voluntary or public health agencies, and nearly 25% of home health care agencies are hospital-based (National Association of Home Care, 1998; Estes et al., 1993).

Agencies may specialize in providing high-tech services or be primarily devoted to providing homemaker/chore services (Dey, 1996). They may focus on one type of home care service (i.e., skilled nursing) or a combination of services (i.e., skilled nursing and hospice). Those agencies that are Medicare-certified represent primarily the skilled nursing segment of the industry. They do not capture the full range of services provided in the home and the multitude of providers, formal and informal, who provide the care. Noncertified agencies may be involved primarily in homemaker-home health aide services (20%), hospice and/or bereavement services (25%), high-tech services (13%), or several different services (42%) (National Association for Home Care, 1995).

TABLE 2.1 Number of Home Health and Hospice Agencies, Current Patients and Discharges: United States, 1992, 1994, and 1996

Type of estimate	1992	1994	1996
Agencies	8,000	10,900	13,500
Current patients	1,284,200	1,950,400	2,486,800
Discharges	3,273,300	5,600,200	8,169,900

Source: Haupt, B. J. (1998b).

HOME CARE USE AND TRENDS

Recent Trends in Home Health and Hospice Care

Recent analyses from the 1996 National Survey of Home and Hospital Care permit the examination of national trends from 1992 to 1996 (Haupt, 1998a). The data are limited in that they do not reflect the diversity in the field but do show the dramatic growth over these 4 years alone in the numbers of home health care agencies and hospices, and clients served. Table 2.1 shows that as of 1996, there were 2.5 million current patients and 8.2 million discharges from 13,500 accredited home health and hospice care agencies in the United States. The number of discharges alone nearly tripled in this short time period (Haupt, 1998a). In 1996 the majority of the agencies (86%) were providing home health care services, whereas the remainder focused on providing hospice services (Haupt, 1998b). Of those agencies providing home health care services, 83% were Medicare-certified and 81% were certified under Medicaid (Haupt, 1998a). Eight percent were not certified by either Medicare nor Medicaid. (A more detailed examination of hospice is provided in chapter 5.)

The proliferation of home care is best exemplified by the growth of Medicare-certified agencies. Federal health policy changes have shortened hospital stays, liberalized the Medicare home and health care benefit to make it more accessible to the nation's older population, and allowed greater participation of proprietary home health care agencies (National Association for Home Care, 1995; Rabin & Stockton, 1987). These changes have led to a greater demand for home health care services as well as a substantial increase in the number of visits per episode of care. For example, in 1983, 47 elderly persons per 1,000 Medicare enrollees received home care services. Each person could expect to receive, on average, 27 visits per episode requiring home care (Altman & Walden, 1993). By 1996, the number of persons per 1,000 served had nearly doubled, and the average number of visits per person had increased to 72 (U.S. General Accounting Office, 1997a).

Growth in Home Health Care Services and Costs

The growth in Medicare home health care expenditures is a source of concern for federal policymakers. Medicare, a major funding source, reimburses more than three quarters of the home care claims filed (Hing, 1994). In 1996 Medicare paid $17.7 billion for Part A home health care services and $300 million under Part B (U.S. General Accounting Office, 1997b). As a percent of total Medicare expenditures, home health care spending has risen from 2.4% in 1988 to nearly 9% (Health Care Financing Administration, 1998). (For a more detailed discussion of the growth in Medicare spending for home care, see chapter 1.)

Of particular concern is the skewing of the distribution of visits and the substantial costs for the high users. For example, the percentage of Medicare beneficiaries receiving more than 60 visits per year increased from 10.6% in 1989 to 25.7% in 1993 (U.S. General Accounting Office, 1996). Nearly 11% of Medicare home care recipients had more than 150 visits in 1992. Costs were especially high for this group of heavy users, with an average cost of $17,180 per episode as compared to an average of $2,760 per episode for those who averaged fewer than 150 visits (Vladeck & Miller, 1994).

Characteristics of the Home Care Client

Home care is used by young and old, but elderly consumers represent nearly three quarters of the home care population. Not surprisingly, those age 85 and older utilize home health care in amounts disproportionate to their small population size. They represent less than a quarter of those receiving home care but consume the greatest portion of services delivered (Altman & Walden, 1993). As indicated in Table 2.2, home health care is most likely to be utilized by the elderly (72.2%), women (67.1%), those who are white (65.1%), and those who are widowed (35.3%), as compared to other social statuses.

TABLE 2.2 Percent Distribution of Current Home Health Care Patients, by Selected Demographic Characteristics: United States, 1996

Total Number	Total 2,427,500
	Distribution (%)
Under 45 years	14.3
45–64 years	13.1
65–74 years	21.7
75–84 years	33.8
85 years and older	16.7
Gender	
Male	32.9
Female	67.1
Ethnicity	
White	65.1
Black and other	13.9
Unknown	21.1
Marital status	
Married	29.0
Widowed	35.3
Divorced or separated	4.1
Never married/single	18.7
Unknown	12.8

Source: Haupt, B. J. (1998b).

The home care user is most likely to rely on Medicare or some other public program to pay for home care services (see Table 2.3). Nearly a quarter of the costs for home care is borne by the user via out-of-pocket payments.

Types of Services Provided

As shown in Table 2.4, the most frequent services delivered to home care consumers in 1993 were skilled nursing services (82.8%) and personal care (58.9%). Bathing, dressing, and transferring, as well as light house-

TABLE 2.3 Sources of Payment for Home Care, 1995

Source of payment	Percent
Medicare	48.7
Medicaid	24.2
Private insurance	3.8
Out-of-pocket	22.8
Other and unknown	0.5

Source: National Association for Home Care. (1998).

TABLE 2.4 Percent of Current Elderly Home Health Care Patients 65 Years and Older Who Received Services During the Last 30 Days: United States, 1993[1]

	Total	Male	Female
Total Number	2,622,700	910,500	1,712,220
Percent Distribution (%)			
Skilled nursing services	82.8	86.8	81.1
Personal care[1]	58.9	56.5	59.8
Homemaker/companion services	18.6	14.0	20.6
Physical therapy	17.5	18.8	16.9
Social services	11.5	10.5	11.9
Medications	5.9	4.6	6.4
Durable medical equipment and supplies	4.7	5.9	4.2
Counseling	4.1	4.0	4.1
Continuous home care	3.8	4.9	3.4
Occupational therapy/vocational therapy	3.7	4.1	3.5
Dietary and nutritional services	2.5	2.6	2.5
Speech therapy/audiology	1.3	2.2	1.0
High-tech care	1.2	2.0	0.8

[1]Includes people receiving help in activities of daily living who were not reported as receiving personal care services.

Source: National Home and Hospice Care Survey. (1996).

work, taking medications, and preparing meals, were the types of personal care most often provided. Other home care services commonly used include physical therapy, homemaker and/or companion services, social services, medications, and occupational/vocational therapy. Only about 1% of the elderly population using home care services received high-tech care (e.g., total parenteral nutrition, inhalation therapy; Dey, 1996).

HOME CARE: AN AGE-OLD TRADITION

This brief demographic profile gives only a flavor of the home care industry, the home care client, and the type of services provided. It is important to go beyond these statistics to explore more fully the underlying concepts and models of home care. Home care is not new, but new models of home care delivery have changed the image of home care. Until about a century ago, all health care was provided in the home by family members. But, as medical science and hospital practice played a more prominent role in the organization and delivery of medical care, care in the home was viewed largely as supportive and appropriate when the application of complex medical technology and treatment did not require institutional placement.

As Benjamin (1993) noted, modern medicine has had a profound effect on perceptions of home care as little more than a "residual" service. Two particular concerns of medical practitioners have shaped this misperception. First, medical professionals and insurers suggested that an absence of uniformity and business "deficiencies" could lead to substandard home care. Second, the growing prevalence of chronic illness seemed to compromise the capacity of hospitals; the inability to restore health to the chronically ill in costly hospital settings renewed interest in home care as a viable, and possibly less costly, alternative for this population. Moreover, the multiple needs of those with chronic illness were seen to be a potential "bottomless pit" (Benjamin, 1993, p. 136).

These concerns shaped government and private-sector policies for delivering home care services. Linking modern home care to hospitalization was considered an optimal way to deal with home care "problems" (Benjamin, 1993). Prior hospitalization offered a mechanism to (1) set eligibility and service limitation criteria, (2) involve trained medical personnel, and (3) establish medical protocols for home care. Insurance plans and social welfare programs developed benefit structures that required physicians to prescribe home care following hospitalization and to limit coverage days to assure that the services provided had some rehabilitative or restorative benefit. These requirements effectively restricted home care reimbursement following hospitalization and avoided the amorphous "black hole" of providing care to the chronically ill.

As a result, societal and historical factors were instrumental in the development of the two basic components of modern home care: social supportive services and medical postacute services. Social supportive services are those that are needed to keep the person in the home. They are oriented toward personal care and maintenance of the individual at some level of effective functioning (Rabin & Stockton, 1987). Now, as in the past, however, the provision of these services is largely entrenched in the uncompensated care provided by families and friends. With some exceptions, no special medical knowledge or technical skill is required; therefore, costs per service are lower. These services when provided by health care workers are in high demand by chronically ill persons. They are labor-intensive, and need for services persists over time. And public costs for care can exceed those of institutional care, most particularly for severely dependent persons in need of constant care and supervision (Crawford, Tennstedt, & McKinlay, 1993; Harrow, Tennstedt, & McKinlay, 1995; Kemper, Applebaum, & Harrigan, 1987; Kemper et al., 1988; Kemper & Murtaugh, 1991; U.S. General Accounting Office, 1991). Most of this type of home care is paid out-of-pocket rather than by third-party payers (National Association for Home Care, 1995). However, goals for social supportive services are not well defined, service impacts are not easily observable (e.g., quality of life), and measurement of care outcomes is difficult (Benjamin, 1993).

Medical postacute services may be further classified as intermediate and intensive. When prescribed by physicians, these services are generally provided on a short-term, intermittent basis and largely reimbursable by third-party payers. Postacute goals are grounded in the precepts and standards established by the medical community. Intermediate postacute services are dependent on medical personnel, particularly nurses, but may include care delivered by paraprofessionals and technicians. Intensive postacute services require an extensive use of medical personnel as well as sophisticated technologies in the home setting (Rabin & Stockton, 1987). Postacute services are generally well defined, and outcomes of care (e.g., physical functioning, reduced hospital utilization) are more often than not measurable (Benjamin, 1993).

Social supportive and medical postacute services are integral to the delivery of home care services today. Because each component is inextricably linked with family and medical structures, these home care services are often perceived as two distinct *systems* of home care operating independently of one another. Yet neither component is independent of the other. Home care recipients have multiple needs. As the interplay between medical and social components of home care have become more visible, attention has focused in practice and in research on teasing out the complex relationships that determine who needs home care and what types of home care are given and by whom, as well as the impacts of these factors on outcomes achieved. Specific models of home care have been identified to delineate the boundaries associated with various levels of care.

HOME CARE GOALS AND MODELS

Overall, modern home care providers establish goals that seek to (1) maximize health and functioning of older persons with long-term care needs, (2) support families who care for dependent older persons, (3) enable care recipients to remain in the community, living in the least restrictive environment, and (4) prevent unnecessary use of health care services, especially hospital and nursing home use. The way in which various home care providers operationalize these goals depends in part on the medical and social needs of the people they serve and the outcomes that are likely. For example, the goals and outcomes of an otherwise healthy elderly person who has an infection after hip fracture will be different from those of the frail elderly person in the final stages of a terminal disease. Therefore, in assessing the impact of home care it is important to consider differences in structure, process, and outcomes of care that are pertinent to specific types of home care services. Four distinct models of home care are available. They are high-tech care, hospice, skilled home care, and low-tech custodial care (Hughes, 1992).

Reduced hospital admissions and lengths of stay, as well as technological developments, have played a major role in the emergence of *high-tech home care* models. Infusion pumps and portable dialysis units make it possible to provide intensive medical care that a decade ago could be provided only in hospitals. The home care provider serving the needs of persons with complex medical needs requires specialized expertise to deliver services such as respirator/ventilator therapy, IV antibiotic therapy, chemotherapy, enteral and parenteral nutrition, and renal dialysis (see chapter 3).

The *hospice* model focuses on needs of the terminally ill and his or her family. The goal is to provide palliative rather than curative care. In addition, an emphasis is placed on minimizing the psychological and spiritual pain of the patient and family that is associated with an impending death. A number of different providers, paid and unpaid, skilled and unskilled, may care for the dying person in his or her home. Skilled nursing services, social services, medications, counseling, volunteer services, homemaker-household services, and physician services are the types of services commonly provided (Haupt, 1998b). Support for and use of this model has grown since the 1980s and can expect to be popular with cost-conscious managed care providers (see chapter 5 for further discussion of hospice).

Skilled nursing is the home care model around which Medicare home health benefits are organized (Hughes, 1992). Services provided by the Medicare-certified home health care agency are principally skilled nursing and rehabilitation services (e.g., physical, speech, and occupational therapy). The elderly individual who is eligible for Medicare home care benefits can receive medical and technical assistance in his or her home following a hospitalization. To receive these Medicare benefits, the individual must be homebound, be certified by a physician to be in need of skilled care, and require care on an intermittent or part-time basis. Because the services provided must be determined to be medically necessary, the skilled nursing provider's goal may be to provide services until the client achieves pre-illness functional status or until care can be turned over to a low-tech home care provider. Furthermore, because hospitalization is more common among the elderly than other age groups, the demand for postacute care will continue to be strong. However, as one of the most rapidly increasing cost components of the Medicare program, changes in the structure of the home care benefit are likely to occur.

Low-tech home care is provided primarily to chronically ill or disabled persons and is the model for which the elderly have the greatest need. This type of home care is provided in a number of different types of settings, including domiciliary care, adult foster care, board and care, and assisted living facilities. Estimates of the number of persons who receive this type of home care range anywhere from 600,000 to 1 million older persons (Eckert & Lyon, 1992). The care is custodial in nature.

Paid services are provided primarily by paraprofessionals, who offer assistance with homemaker/chore/housekeeping activities. The focus of care is on improvement or maintenance of functional status. Medicare does not pay for such care, and funding under Medicaid is limited.

Although each of these models is distinct, in practice they are not mutually exclusive. Those who receive services in the home differ and their needs change depending on stage and type of illness, age, and availability of informal support. One episode may require services from a single type of care (e.g., chemotherapy) or different types of care (e.g., chemotherapy and personal care assistance). Services provided in the home may be delivered by multiple providers.

Even with the best efforts, coordinating care across multiple providers and settings is difficult. The interplay between the various models may be acknowledged, but providers, professionals, and nonprofessionals alike can have difficulty recognizing if and when goals conflict (Weiner & Skaggs, 1994).

EXPANDING THE HOME CARE CONCEPT

Current political and market pressures continue to modify home care. There are several key trends affecting the concept of home care (Kane, 1995). Federal policies for confining services only to those with medically prescribed need have constrained states attempting to reduce institutional costs and delay institutional placements. For example, reimbursement regulations that stipulate payment for "medical care services," not "room and board," have lacked the flexibility to accommodate evolving low-tech models that combine housing and services, and stress individual autonomy and the maximization of functioning, as in the case of assisted living. Some states have taken steps to alter these policies, while others are examining these issues critically (Snow, 1995). Welfare reform under the Personal Responsibility and Work Opportunity Reconciliation Act of 1996 has given states greater flexibility in the management and disbursement of resources.

Long-term care is no longer confined to one image of a frail elderly person. It has become more universal in its focus, extending to include all ages, diagnoses, and physical and mental impairments (Office of the Assistant Secretary for Planning and Evaluation, 1994). State home- and community-based services programs have not been developed exclusively for frail elderly populations. Some programs and federal waivers are focused on the distinct needs of others needing long-term care (i.e., developmentally disabled persons and physically impaired younger persons).

Modified programs attempt to focus on the *functional assistance needed* by dependent people living in the community (Kane, 1995). Personal assistance services (PAS), a reflection of the independent living movement, has become a popular concept that broadly refers to any and all forms of assistance (e.g., personal care, assistive devices, environmental adaptations, etc.) that would enable a disabled person to perform activities he or she would perform without the impairment (Office of the Assistant Secretary for Planning and Evaluation, 1994). Recognizing the expressed desire of persons with disabilities to have more choices available and greater input in the process of choosing services, the Health Care Reform debate of 1993 set the tone for state health care reform efforts that are working to develop programs that are more "consumer-centered."

KEEPING THE RESEARCH AGENDA MOVING FORWARD

Our understanding of home care has increased, but there are many more unanswered questions. Past examinations of the use and effectiveness of these services have provided valuable information, but current efforts continue to lack the definitional clarity and the methodological sophistication needed to reveal how the complexities associated with caring for chronically ill persons influence home care outcomes (Ory & Duncker, 1992). Research in this area has suffered from accepted methods and limited databases. Home care continues to be viewed in research either as a monolithic entity or in simplistic dichotomies (e.g., acute vs. long-term, medical vs. social, informal vs. formal, etc.). There has been a failure to identify the essential components of home care, making it difficult to point to select processes that will produce intended benefits. There are a number of outcomes for home care that are relevant to those served. Yet, possibly in response to budgetary and policy interests, research in this area has focused unduly on costs. In setting a course for future research that will ultimately inform on the nature and effectiveness of home care delivery systems, it is necessary to highlight relevant themes, old and new, and to point out the challenges that can be expected in tackling research in this area.

First, studies of home care must continue to untangle the complexities associated with caring for chronically ill persons and the heterogeneity of the population served. Research studies in this area must describe how distinct models of home care interact and change in practice. Condition-specific variations within the home care population have important implications for how care is planned, delivered, and responded to by subpopulations on the basis of age, race, and ethnicity. Home care is a blending of formal, informal, social, and medical features. Recognition of how these features blend or remain distinct enables examinations of processes that yield a positive or negative outcome within a specific group. Home care must be examined in relation to its linkages with the acute and long-term care systems. More explicit conceptualizations of particular home care services (e.g., in-home respite care) are needed to probe factors associated with patterns of use to develop a more in-depth comprehension of how and why these services affect client and caregiver well-being and their use of institutional and community-based services. Understanding how formal providers interact with informal providers and investigating how transitions in acute and long-term care influence or are influenced by these relationships is critical. (See chapter 4 for a more detailed discussion.)

Second, the intricacies of home care in its broadest sense can only be understood in the context in which services are provided. Differentiating home care provided in a person's own home, a board and care home, or as a set of services within a continuing care retirement community provides important insights on the populations served and resources available to subpopulations. This, in turn, has important implications for identifying and examining how setting characteristics may facilitate or constrain the provision of care. Studies in this regard may also provide important information about factors that contribute to the frequency of transitions in care and the outcomes associated.

Third, the impact of home care should not be reduced to whether or not this type of service is an appropriate substitute for institutional placement. Models of home care assume distinct goals and outcomes that are reasonable given the nature and complexity of the situation in which services are provided. Theoretical frameworks for examining the effectiveness of home care are crucial. In measuring the effectiveness of home care, research must examine the degree to which goals, professional and client-directed, are achieved. Studies must specify the type, intensity, and frequency of services delivered. They must identify and examine the pathways that link various services to specific outcomes.

Finally, studies of home care must continue to examine how current market and policy trends are changing the sector. Important research questions emerge. To what extent are biosocial views of health care incorporated in various home care models, and how do outcomes compare to more traditional systems of home care delivery? How will interdisciplinary teams interact with home care providers and clients, and how will these interactions affect quality of care, worker satisfaction, and the client's quality of life? How will managed care providers use home care systems to meet the needs of special populations? Will managed care arrangements alter the way in which home care is provided? If so, how will these changes affect clients and their providers? In a health care policy environment that stresses quality improvement, how will standards for home care providers change? How will home care quality be measured by state policymakers and managed care providers? How will these requirements affect specific model types and the home care industry in general?

CONCLUSION

On a final note, the reconceptualization of long-term care reflects some important trends that are and will continue to change the way home care is delivered. Maintaining the long-term care consumer in the community requires a biosocial view of health care that recognizes the medical and social components of home care. A life course perspective will have to be an integral aspect of assessing long-term care needs and services. Therefore, in developing care plans for the home care client, the home care provider must be cognizant of the person's short-term and long-term care needs. Multidisciplinary interaction and cooperation under the rubric of "case management" will remain an important focus. The team approach has the potential of individualizing care, empowering the consumer, and providing reasonable assurances that specific care goals do not compromise overall care goals. Home care providers will be required to consult with the team and act in accordance with goals stipulated by the team. Importantly, the gatekeeping function of the multidisciplinary team offers a mechanism for managed care providers to seek greater efficiencies in service utilization. In addition, state long-term care programs and waivers that continue to deemphasize provider control may have the benefit of creating greater consumer control and autonomy over the care provided in the community.

There remains uncertainty about the degree to which consumer autonomy and choice will be reflected in developing programs. The home care provider may face significant challenges in delivering care to clients. Moreover, these challenges may change depending on whether program philosophies are consumer-directed or consumer-centered. Most importantly, advancing technology and evolving supportive living arrangements will continue to affect the way in which home care services are provided to noninstitutionalized elderly. *Home care,* even as we know it today, may become a misnomer.

REFERENCES

Altman, B., & Walden, D. (1993, April). *Home health care: Use, expenditures, and source of payment* (AHCPR Pub. No. 93-0040). National Medical Expenditure Survey Research Findings 15, Agency for Health Care Policy Research. Rockville, MD: Public Health Service.

American Association of Homes and Services for the Aging. (1997). *Linking housing and health services for older persons.* New York: Milbank Memorial Fund.

Benjamin, A. E. (1992). An overview of in-home health and supportive services for older persons. In M. G. Ory & A. P. Duncker (Eds.), *In-home care for older people: Health and supportive services* (pp. 9–52). Newbury Park, CA: Sage.

_____. (1993). An historical perspective on home care policy. *Milbank Quarterly, 71,* 129–166.

Bringewatt, R. (1995). *Integrating care for people with chronic conditions.* Bloomington, MN: National Chronic Care Consortium.

Cohen, R. A., & Van Nostrand, J. F. (1995). *Trends in the health of older Americans: United States, 1994.* National Center for Health Statistics. *Vital Health Statistics 3*(30).

Crawford, S. L., Tennstedt, S. L., & McKinlay, J. B. (1993). *Substitution of formal and informal care in the elderly.* Presented at the 1993 American Statistical Association Winter Conference, January 3–5.

Dey, A. N. (1996). *Characteristics of elderly home health care users: Data from the 1993 National Home and Hospice Care Survey* (Advance Data from the Vital and Health Statistics of the Centers for Disease Control and Prevention, No. 272). Hyattsville, MD: National Center for Health Statistics, U.S. Department of Health and Human Services.

Eckert, J. K., & Lyon, S. M. (1992). Board and care homes: From the margins to the mainstream in the 1990s. In M. G. Ory & A. P. Duncker (Eds.), *In-home care for older people: Health and supportive services* (pp. 97–114). Newbury Park, CA: Sage.

Estes, C. L., Swan J. H., & associates. (1993). *The long term care crisis: Elders trapped in the no-care zone.* Newbury Park, CA: Sage.

Harrow, B. S., Tennstedt, S. L., & McKinlay, J. B. (1995). How costly is it to care for disabled elders in a community setting? *Gerontologist, 35,* 803–813.

Haupt, B. J. (1998a). *An overview of home health and hospice care patients: 1996 National Home and Hospice Care Survey* (Advance Data from the Vital and Health Statistics of the Centers for Disease Control and Prevention, No. 297). Hyattsville, MD: National Center for Health Statistics, U.S. Department of Health and Human Services.

_____. (1998b). *Characteristics of hospice care users: 1996 National Home and Hospice Care Survey* (Advance Data from Vital and Health Statistics of the Centers for Disease Control and Prevention, No. 299). Hyattsville, MD: National Center for Health Statistics, U.S. Department of Health and Human Services.

Health Care Financing Administration. (1998). *A profile of Medicare: Chartbook, 1998.* Washington, DC: U.S. Department of Health and Human Services.

Hing, E. (1994). *Characteristics of elderly home health patients: Preliminary data from the 1992 National Home and Hospice Care Survey* (Advance Data from Vital and Health Statistics of the National Centers for Disease Control and Prevention, No. 247). Hyattsville, MD: National Center for Health Statistics, U.S. Department of Health and Human Services.

Hughes, S. L. (1992). Home care: Where we are and where we need to go. In M. G. Ory & A. P. Duncker (Eds.), *In-home care for older people: Health and supportive services* (pp. 53–74). Newbury Park, CA: Sage.

Kane, R. A. (1995). Expanding the home care concept: Blurring distinctions among home care, institutional care, and other long-term care services. *Milbank Quarterly, 73,* 161–185.

Kane, R. A., Kane, R. L., & Ladd, R. C. (1998). *The heart of long-term care.* New York: Oxford University Press.

Kassner, E., & Bectel, R. W. (1998). *Midlife and older Americans with disabilities: Who gets help?* (AARP Chartbook). Washington, DC: American Association of Retired Persons.

Kemper, P., Applebaum, R., & Harrigan, M. (1987). Community-based care demonstrations: What have we learned? *Health Care Financing Review, 8*(4), 87–100.

Kemper, P. R., Brown, R. S., Carcagno, G. J., Applebaum, R. A., Christianson, J. B., Corson, W., Dunstan, S. M., Grannemann, T., Harrigan, M., Holden, N., Phillips, B. R., Schore, J., Thornton, C., Wooldridge, J., & Skidmore, F. (1988). The evaluation of the national long-term care demonstration [Special issue]. *Health Services Research, 23*(1).

Kemper, P., & Murtaugh, C. M. (1991). Lifetime use of nursing home care. *New England Journal of Medicine, 324,* 595–600.

Manton, K. G., Corder, L., Stallard, E. (1997). Chronic disability trends in the U.S. elderly population, 1982–1994. *Proceedings of the National Academy of Sciences, 94,* 2593–2598.

Manton, K. G., Stallard, E., & Corder, L. (1995). Changes in morbidity and chronic disability in the U.S. elderly population: Evidence from the 1982, 1984 and 1989 National Long-term Care Survey. *Journals of Gerontology: Social Science,* (July), S194–S204.

National Association for Home Care. (1995). *Basic statistics about home care,* 1994 (information sheet). Washington, DC: Author.

———. (1998). *Basic statistics about home care,* 1997 (information sheet). Washington, DC: Author.

National Home and Hospice Care Survey. (1996). (Advance Data from Vital and Health Statistics of the Centers for Disease Control and Prevention, No. 272.) Hyattsville, MD: National Center for Health Statistics, U.S. Department of Health and Human Services.

Office of the Assistant Secretary for Planning and Evaluation. (1994). *Background paper on personal assistance services and related reports.* (Office of Disability, Aging and Long Term Care Policy, November 2). Washington, DC: U.S. Department of Health and Human Services.

Ory, M. G., & Duncker, A. P. (Eds.). (1992). *In-home care for older people: Health and supportive services.* Newbury Park, CA: Sage.

Rabin, D. L., & Stockton, P. (1987). *Long-term care for the elderly: A factbook.* New York: Oxford University Press.

Saucier, P., & Riley, T. (1994). *Managing care for beneficiaries of Medicaid and Medicare: Prospects and pitfalls.* Portland, ME: National Academy for State Health Policy.

Snow, K. I. (1995). *State long term care programs at a glance.* Portland, ME and Waltham, MA: The Center for Vulnerable Populations, a collaboration of the National Academy for State Health Policy and the Institute for Health Policy, Brandeis University.

Stone, R. I. (1995, June). *Long-term care policy in the United States.* Paper presented at U.S.–Italy Conference on Long-Term Care, National Institutes of Health, Bethesda, MD.

U.S. Bureau of the Census (1996). *65+ in the United States*. Current Population Reports, Special Studies, P23-190. Washington, DC: U.S. Government Printing Office.

_____. (1997). *Aging in the United States–past, present and future*. Washington, DC: U.S. Government Printing Office.

U.S. General Accounting Office. (1991). *Long-term care: Projected needs of the aging baby boom generation* (Report to the Chairman, Special Committee on Aging, U.S. Senate, June). Washington, DC: U.S. Government Printing Office.

_____. (1996). *Medicare: Home health utilization expands while program controls deteriorate* (Report to the Chairman, Special Committee on Aging, U.S. Senate, March). Washington, DC: U.S. Government Printing Office.

_____. (1997a). *Medicare post-acute care: Home health and skilled nursing facility cost growth and proposals for prospective payment* (statement of William J. Scanlon, director, Health Financing and Systems Issues, Health, Education and Human Services Division, March 4). Washington, DC: U.S. Government Printing Office.

_____. (1997b). *Medicare home health agencies: Certification process ineffective in excluding problem agencies* (Report to the Special Committee on Aging, U.S. Senate, December). Washington, DC: U.S. Government Printing Office.

Vladeck, B. C., & Miller, N. A. (1994). The Medicare home health initiative. *Health Care Financing Review, 16*(1), 7–15.

Waidmann, T., & Manton, K. (1998). International evidence on disability trends among the elderly. Washington, DC: Office of the Assistant Secretary for Planning and Evaluation, U.S. Department of Health and Human Services.

Weiner, J. P., & Skaggs, J. (1994). *Current approaches to integrating acute and long-term care financing and services*. Washington, DC: American Association of Retired Persons, Public Policy Institute.

SECTION TWO

THE PROVISION OF HOME CARE

CHAPTER 3

The Use of Technology in Home Care

Leighton E. Cluff
Patricia Flatley Brennan

"[T]he high-tech home care industry has rapidly and relentlessly erased, for increasing numbers of families, the boundaries between hospital and home, between intensive care units and the living room" (Arras, 1994, p. S1). Acutely ill, chronically ill, disabled, and impaired persons—once cared for only in hospitals and other institutions—can remain in their homes because technology-based home care is now possible. Indeed, some technology-dependent persons can have sufficient improved function to make it possible for them to return to work and to a more normal life (Smith, 1994).

Contributing to the rapid expansion of technology-based home care have been medical technology designed for use in the home, readily available communication technologies to enhance home care, rising costs of hospital care, reduction of capacity in acute and long-term care facilities, and the preferences of those who are sick to be cared for in the community rather than in institutions (Larkins & Hellige, 1992). Health problems of growing numbers of aging Americans, longer survival of severely impaired infants and adults, and the emergence of innovative therapies to treat or ameliorate previously incurable diseases have also contributed to a growing demand for use of medical technologies in the home. In addition, the use of complex medical technologies in the home has been encouraged by greater public and private insurance coverage for these interventions.

A variety of simple measures can enable disabled persons to live at home and care for themselves. More sophisticated and complex technologies permit home-based interventions, promoting self-care and active participation by patients and families in patient management. Increasingly available information technology enables frail and disabled persons to gain ready access to health care professionals who can provide advice and help. Medical technologies adapted for home use and information systems and technology are critically important in the provision of home care (Weinstein, 1993).

Home care for persons requiring innovative, even life-supporting, medical technology is a reality in England, France, Sweden, Japan, and other industrialized countries, as well as in the United States. France, for example, has had extensive experience providing mechanical ventilation in the home for patients with chronic respiratory insufficiency, including data information systems to evaluate patient outcomes. Diffusion of these technologies for the benefit of all persons requires changes in the manner in which both professionals and laypersons interact in the health care system (Goldberg, 1989; Weinstein, 1993).

In the United States, technologies to support home care of persons with acute and chronic illnesses range from simple modification of the home environment to complex medical devices such as respirators and infusion systems. Few studies of the use of high-tech home care (information and medical technologies) have been published, in part because few coordinated systems of hospital and community-based home care services, providing data and information on home care within the context of all health care services, have been developed. Research will be required to evaluate the impact of high-tech home care on patients, families, and society, as well as on hospitals, nursing homes, and other segments of health care services. Similarly, education and training strategies for new and existing health professionals, along with the efficient design of organizations to coordinate technology-based home care services, depend on the availability of reliable data and information derived from model programs. This chapter attempts to address some of these issues.

THE TECHNOLOGY OF HOME CARE

Technologies of interest in the home-care of ill persons and their family caregivers fall into three general areas: (1) straightforward application of known engineering and ergonomic principles that promote safety, (2) skillful application of medical devices, and (3) appropriate application of information technologies (Parker & Thorslund, 1991). Each provides benefits that depend, in part, on the extent to which the patient or family caregiver is able to make appropriate use of the technology.

Engineering and Ergonomic Improvements

Simple changes in households offer great assistance in promoting safety. Removal of environmental impediments and installation of simple technical aids make it possible for many impaired persons to remain in their homes (Parker & Thorslund,1991). Safe flooring, canes and railings, wide hallways and doorways, ramps rather than steps, grab bars in bathtubs and showers, amplification of sound in audio equipment, visual aids, and enlargement of lettering on bottles and boxes, among other similar efforts and devices, can materially help disabled persons to remain functionally effective at home. Most often these aids are put in place by the impaired person or family members, but guidance from others, particularly occupational therapists, can be of great value.

Medical Technology

The increasing use of medical technology in home care places demands on families and on health care professionals in ways not known a decade or more ago. A survey of home care agencies in California indicated that 15.3% of patients required high-technology nursing care (White & Smith, 1993). As the number of severely ill and disabled persons requiring such technology increases, families and health professionals are assuming responsibilities in the home that might previously have been considered impossible. For example, the high cost of cardiac care and the increasing number of patients with cardiac disease make medical and nursing care at home an attractive alternative to costly institutional care. The latest advances in medicine and technology are transforming cardiac home care, decreasing trips to and from the clinic and hospital (Lenane, 1994). Home care professionals are conducting advanced cardiac assessments and caring for patients at home with chronic refractory heart failure requiring intensive medical management (Sherman, 1995).

Examples of complex technology now employed for care of persons in their homes provide only a glimmer of what is available and cannot come close to predicting what will become available for home care in the near and distant future. Parenteral and enteral infusion of medications, including agents to alleviate pain (morphine), and of antibiotic and nutritional products, is growing so rapidly that industries have been established to oversee and direct infusion therapy (Ross-Degnan et al., 1995; Sheldon & Bender, 1994; Williams, 1994). Careful patient selection and careful preparation and training of patient and family caregiver are important to avoid untoward events such as infection (Sherman, 1995). Hemodialysis in the home for those with chronic renal impairment has increased ever since federal legislation provided financing for this care through Medicare. Mechanical ventilation as a life-sustaining device is available for use in the home, but this technology presents problems of safety and efficacy, in the same way as other complex technology. Increasing numbers of patients cared for at home with refractory and chronic heart failure require intensive medical management and follow-up by nurses trained in advanced cardiac assessment and care. The patient or family caregiver, if available, must assume responsibility for use of this and other technology, whereas, in the hospital, use of technology is the responsibility of professionally trained persons. Moreover, physicians regularly oversee use of complex technology in the hospital, but rarely in the home, even though recent studies indicate the importance of the physician in overseeing care in the home as part of a system of patient care.

Boundaries between hospitals, nursing homes, and community care make it difficult if not impossible to provide patients and families with integrated, coordinated, and seamless health care services. These boundaries must be decreased or eliminated if home care and other segments of health care are to reach their full potential in improving patients' lives and possibly reducing the cost associated with institutional care (Bingley, 1993).

Information Technology

Information technology plays several key roles in home care: (1) ensuring communication among professional providers, (2) facilitating providers' communication with patients and families, (3) assessing the quality of care in the home, and (4) providing data for management of resources—personnel and financial (Brennan, Moore, & Smyth, 1995; Brennan & Ripich, 1994).

Electronic systems for communication between patient and provider are increasingly important in providing home care. The development of reliable telecommunications technology enables caregivers, patients, and management to access health information. Excessive nursing time spent in paper documentation is arguably the single biggest business problem facing home care agencies, and reliable information technology can materially remedy this problem (Braunstein, 1993). Computer networks, telephone message services, and other initiatives provide home care nurses unique opportunities to reach patients and families with information about health promotion, disease prevention, and illness management.

A project known as ComputerLink provided homebound persons access to information, communication, and decision-support tools. Two ComputerLinks were developed, one serving persons with AIDS (Brennan & Ripich, 1994), a second supporting the caregivers of persons with Alzheimer's disease (Brennan et al., 1995). Placing the ComputerLink in the context of other telecommunications-based services provided information about using these services in home care. A nurse-moderator made initial visits to each patient to assess needs and provided training in the use of the ComputerLink system. Information was designed to enhance self-management, promote effective home-based treatment of patients, and promote caregiver understanding of illness-specific issues (Bass, McClendon, Brennan, & McCarthy, 1998). Access to the system was through (1) a bulletin board for information; (2) electronic mail (e-mail) through which users could send messages or receive answers to inquiries; and (3) the posting of questions posed by users, which were useful in ensuring that all providers were equally informed. ComputerLink was the first project demonstrating that computer networks could be customized to address the home health care needs of chronically ill patients and caregivers.

Over a 4-year period, the ComputerLink project had 15,000 user accesses, averaging about 10 to 13 minutes per log-on. Generally, users accessed the system twice a day (24-hour periods). Most encounters were between 10:00 P.M. and 3:00 P.M. Users reported that ComputerLink served as a "support system without walls" for homebound patients with AIDS and caregivers of patients with Alzheimer's disease (Brennan et al., 1995; Brennan & Ripich, 1994).

There are several other examples of innovative information technology systems in home care. For instance, the Comprehensive Health Evaluation and Social Support project (CHESS) uses a client-server model to implement disease-specific counseling and support services (Gustafson et al., 1999). Like ComputerLink, CHESS provides home care support to ill persons, but is directed to women concerned about or actually in treatment for breast cancer and persons with AIDS, and is now expanding to address the needs of persons with substance abuse problems and heart disease. CHESS is a freestanding system, not a special set of services within a larger network. It provides graphics and sound, but it requires a more complex and expensive personal computer platform than does ComputerLink.

Other community-based telecommunications efforts make use of telephones. Telepractice (Alemi et al., 1996) uses a voice-telephone platform to provide social support and clinical management for women in high-risk pregnancies. It has been expanded to assist visiting nurses to care for persons with chronic cardiac disease. Lindberg (1997) and colleagues reported the use of two-way television linkage between home and clinic, allowing patients a daily "videovisit" for health promotion, disease management, and medication checks. Health Maintenance Organizations (HMOs) have begun to offer telephone-triage and Internet connections for education and patient assistance (Kastens, 1998).

In short, computer networks serve as convenient and efficient vehicles for delivering nursing services to patients at home. Such networks provide supervised information, decision support, and communication services to homebound patients. Electronic communications can provide patient support and an emergency response system. Computer networks represent an ideal technology for the delivery of certain nursing services to the home.

The benefits of this technology to nurses and patients they care for are numerous (Braunstein, 1993). Nurses can access patients in an efficient and supportive manner. They can respond to multiple levels of need for their patients. They can attend to emotional as well as medical nursing needs. They can use the system at a time, frequency, and duration of their choice.

Computer networks also provide support to patients caring for themselves and reduce their sense of isolation, while supporting family caregivers as well.

The ability of nurses to assess a situation in the home and initiate appropriate interventions can be enhanced by computer technology (Alter, 1994; Ripich, Moore, & Brennan, 1992). Computer networks can provide data links with hospitals, physician offices, clinics, and community health centers. Charting of patient records by computer can provide more comprehensive documentation and better patient management (Gogola, 1995). Electronic systems can improve productivity, increase home care revenue, and reduce billing errors for providers and agencies. Management of nursing information provides a means to better allocate human and financial resources (Braunstein, 1993).

Providers of home care and their patients do require training before computer technology can be fully embraced as a way to improve home care services (Brennan & Ripich, 1994; O'Leary, Mann, & Perkash, 1991). Training programs for providers in computer-based instruction, computerized monitoring of trainee progress, on-line tutorial support, and computerized test administration and marketing have proved to be useful (Kenny & Murray, 1993).

PROVIDERS AND RECIPIENTS OF HOME CARE

Home care is provided mostly by people with no special training in medicine, nursing, or the use of complex technology (see chapter 4). Health professionals, however, are crucial to the assessment of patient need, providing services and overseeing and monitoring the use of technology in the home. Physician involvement is especially important in prescribing and overseeing technology-based home care (Power, 1995).

Health care increasingly is a world of technology, and all who are responsible for and provide home care must know and understand technologic services for those at home. They also must know that managing the technology is not enough; *caring* for the patient is essential (Lindeman, 1992).

Health Professionals

Nurses are more deeply involved than other professionals in providing home care and in the use of home care technology. They have special responsibilities for patients and their families who must be involved in the use of high-tech equipment and procedures in the home, throughout each day and night, when the nurse is there intermittently (Handy, 1989; Zwolski, 1989). Nurses provide for and monitor the use of technology in home care. They must be involved in the careful selection of patients for whom the use of technology in home care is appropriate, and in the training of patients and families (Hill, 1995; Sherman, 1995). Critical care clinical nurse specialists have an increasingly important role in the use of complex medical technology in the home (Roe-Prior, Watts, & Burke, 1994). Indeed, they should be prepared for involvement in hospital discharge planning, as well as in practice in home care. These nurses also serve as consultants to home care agencies, provide training for patients and families, and assist in hospital-to-home coordination.

"Many authorities agree on the key role played by physicians—not only in assuring the medical necessity of care, but also in promoting the integration of medical and social services as well as acute and long-term care. However, some lament the fact that many physicians seem to do little more than routinely 'rubber stamp' the plans of care prepared by home health agency staff" (National Health Policy Forum, 1996, p. 7). Physicians, generally, are not well informed about the circumstances, difficulties, and risks, as well as the potential benefits, of technology in home care. In fact, physicians often have dissociated themselves from many of the responsibilities and potential risks associated with home care (Arras, 1995). Indeed, many physicians do not make home visits, and home care agencies, generally, are dissatisfied with physicians' lack of involvement.

Areas where physicians could benefit from home care involvement are improvement of home care clinical skills, knowledge of home care technology, and the usefulness and problems of medical technology in the home (Keenan, Hepburn, Ripsin, Webster, & Bland, 1992). Physicians may appreciate the importance of home health care and its burgeoning technology, but some have doubts about its expansion and appropriate use in the home (Champlin, 1989). With the anticipated continuing growth of sophisticated technology that can be used for home care, physicians must understand the potentially unlimited spectrum of home care products and services (Bernstein, Hankwitz, & Portnow, 1990; Willging, 1995).

Patients and Families

Patients' homes are their private domain, and care in this setting cannot be appropriately equated with care in institutions. This presents a challenge for all who provide home care (Liaschenko, 1994). To care for the patient and entire family, home care providers need to be sensitive to the characteristics of the community in which the patient and family reside, the structure of family relationships, patient and family expectations from care at home, and the ability of the patient and family to physically and emotionally manage the technology and care of the patient (Handy, 1989).

Greater participation by the patient and caregiver in development and implementation of a treatment plan helps the patient and family to remain intact and committed (Sheldon & Bender, 1994). Otherwise, stress can be significant, at times overbearing (Smith, Geiffer, & Bieker, 1991; Smith, Moushey, Ross, & Geiffer, 1993). Family member relationships and roles often change when a patient becomes technologically dependent. When families and other nonprofessional caregivers are prepared for their responsibilities and receive appropriate support from home care nurses and other health professionals, they can adapt and be capable and effective (Smith et al., 1991). Members of a family, or friends, who assume care responsibilities for a technology-dependent person in the home may experience anxiety, frustration, and depression. In some instances, this can lead to conflict and desperation, family disruption and disintegration. The nurse is essential in helping these caregivers.

It is possible to reduce the duration of hospitalization for patients (e.g., those who have undergone a total hip replacement) by the provision of planned physical therapy in the home (Moller, Goldie, & Jonsson, 1992). Pharmacists, physical therapists, dentists, podiatrists, medical social workers, clinical psychologists, and others are now involved in home care, and will be more involved as use of newer technology and different types of professional services are required in the home setting. Education and training programs for all health professionals, particularly nurses, must prepare them for their particular and special roles in home care, *including* support of patients and families (Kwan & Anderson, 1991). The increasing number of different health professionals that may be involved in the care of a patient at home also creates considerable demand for regular communication among the professional care providers, and between providers and patients and their family caregivers. A communication system or network, as discussed above, can provide the glue necessary to establish and maintain a seamless system and improve the quality of care (Boling & Keenan, 1992).

SOCIAL AND POLICY ISSUES

Economics of Home Care

In addition to the extraordinary development of sophisticated technology that can be used for care in the home, economics has been a factor in the increased use of high technology in home care. As indicated in other chapters in this volume, health care costs and expenditures have risen greatly over the past few decades. Partly for this reason, health care has moved into alternative settings, including home care; the home has been adapted to provide technology that before was provided only in the hospital or other institutional setting (Sadock, 1995).

> One of the causes of the recent expansion of home care has been the development of revolutionary new medical technology which allows the delivery at home of care which only a few years ago could have been delivered only in a hospital.... Technology has been developed that permits patients to be monitored without the physical presence of a health care professional. The prospects are good for further development of such technology, which, with the added impetus of managed-care, is certain to boost pressures for fewer hospital admissions and increased use of home care, possibly delivered more often by technicians than clinicians. (National Health Policy Forum, 1996, pp. 10–11)

The expectation has been that the use of technology for care in the home will be less costly than care provided in an institution. A number of publications suggest that home care of patients who are dependent on medical technology reduces the costs of care that otherwise would be provided in institutional settings (Arno, Bonuck, & Padgug, 1995; Sheldon & Bender, 1994; Sherman, 1995; Smith, 1994; Williams, 1994; Willging, 1995). Yet ongoing research is needed to adequately document that this is the case (see chapter 9). Patients usually prefer being cared for at home rather than in an institution. Evidence that home care may be less costly than institutional care would accelerate this trend.

The care and support of technology-dependent persons at home can impose considerable financial responsibility on patients, families, communities, states, and the nation. Modification of dwellings to accommodate those who are dependent on different technologies can be a significant expense. Private insurance, Medicare, and Medicaid may assume some of the cost for the technology or equipment necessary for some patients, but copayments often are required, creating difficult financial burdens for patients and families. In those instances where families or other informal caregivers are unavailable, constant or frequent care can be required of health professionals. The cost of constant professional care may not be covered by insurance for as long as is necessary, and in these instances patients and families may become impoverished by paying for it out-of-pocket. Impoverishment can be followed by dependency upon state (Medicaid) support, further burdening public resources.

With the increased use of sophisticated, complex medical technology in the home, studies are needed to evaluate the cost effectiveness and efficacy of this form of home care, contrasted with care in institutional settings. Evaluation of the economic impact of technology-based home care should include attention to the improvement or decline in productivity experienced by family caregivers. This adds an important dimension to the analysis of economic productivity and societal return obtained by home care (Ross-Degnan et al., 1995). (For a more detailed discussion of the costs of home care, see chapter 7. For discussions of the economics of long-term care, more generally, see Binstock, 1998; Meiners, 1996.)

Ethical and Legal Issues

Home health care providers are increasingly faced with ethical dilemmas. The evolution of technology, funding allocation guidelines, and patients requiring more complex care influence the delivery of services, creating both legal and ethical issues (Arras & Dubler, 1994). Nurses providing home health care usually must practice independently, and the possibility that they may not be adequately prepared to make ethical decisions makes their task difficult. Interestingly, a study has indicated that the most common ethical problems faced by nurses are difficulties with payer regulations and the competency of health care workers (Haddad, 1992).

As life-sustaining technology is used in the home, dying in the home with caring families and friends may increase, and dying in a hospital will correspondingly decrease. Death-denying attitudes and an inability to cope with a dying family member, too often result in the hospitalization of dying patients. An emphasis on useless rescue interventions can influence professionals to remove dying patients from their home, even when the family may wish for the patient to die at home. Here is a situation, however, where health professionals, nurses in particular, are in an important position to assist families and patients in accepting the inevitability of death and the desirability of patients dying in the presence of loved ones. However, "[a]lthough family members might have good reasons to choose the option of dying at home for themselves and their loved ones, the possible long-range consequences should be part of their decision calculus" (Arras & Dubler, 1995, p. 3).

It has been suggested that home care ethics committees, possibly developed by home care agencies, could formulate appropriate guidelines for the use of life-sustaining interventions in the home (Abel, 1990; deBlois, 1994). However, as Arras and Dubler (1995) have asked, regarding high-tech home care:

> "What kinds of homes and families do we want our society to foster, and at what price?" Our problem is thus better described not as an ethical "dilemma," but as a complex social phenomenon that improves life for many, while threatening to erode for others the conditions that tend to foster important social goods and opportunities—such as a nurturing home life with its intimacy, privacy, and freedom from bureaucratic and rationalized trappings of institutions.... (p. 4)

The increase in technologically sophisticated home care services challenges individual patients and family members to examine their preferences for life support and life-sustaining technologies. The establishment of advanced directives—a living will or a health care power of attorney—has been helpful for this purpose. Individuals, particularly the elderly, are urged to execute advance directives in which they state their personal wishes about the use of life-restoring or life-prolonging diagnostic and therapeutic procedures and interventions if they are faced with terminal illness. Awareness of patient and family wishes, as expressed in living wills, can help providers identify procedures, interventions, and technology that are proscribed by the patient and family. However, too few patients and families make choices and prepare advance directives. Home care providers and agencies are in a position to encourage and assist them in this process. States usually have forms available that can be used for advance directives, based on state statutes. Often, these forms can be modified to suit an individual's preferences. Providers (especially nurses) can help individuals and their families to understand how advance directives can be designed to meet particular cultural, religious, and other circumstances. These efforts can also enhance the relationships that evolve between the nurse, patient, and family (Marren, 1993).

Although present and future technology for home use may improve patient quality of life and outcomes, and possibly decrease health care costs, it can also, on occasion, result in adverse consequences, affecting patients, families, and providers of care. The probability of adverse consequences could be reduced through a clearer delineation of the role that physicians should assume in prescribing, directing, and monitoring high-tech home care, and working with other health care providers. If this is not done and implemented, nurses and home care agencies will have to assume responsibilities that traditionally belong to physicians, as already is happening (Portnow, 1994). Overall, too little is known about the beneficial and adverse impacts of high-technology home care on individuals, families, and social and economic conditions.

Adverse consequences sometimes give rise to legal issues; as a consequence, many publications and manuals on the law and home care are available (e.g., see Nathanson, 1996). In the current social and legal climate nurses are increasingly subject to litigation. The increased professional standing of nursing and the greater role of nurses in decision-making aspects of home health care are largely responsible for this. There are risks in providing care in the home or elsewhere, and this is intensified by the expanding use of complex medical technology in home care, where the nurse may have responsibility not shared by physicians or other health professionals. Claims of negligence against nurses relate mostly to patient injury. Nurses who practice independently are at considerable personal risk, as contrasted with their risk in claims of negligence in hospitals, when the hospital itself may be the object of the litigation. Home care agencies employing home care nurses, however, also may be liable to claims of negligence. There have been some interesting recent legal cases involving issues of liability in the use of technology in home care, but the cumulative case law does not as yet provide systematic guidance. In addition, the use of technology in homes has opened up some state licensure issues, such as the rights of nurses and physicians to interact electronically across state lines.

Factors predisposing to legal risk in home care can be defined. Risk management concepts and strategies should be developed to assist nurses and home care agencies in recognizing intrinsic danger or risk and reduce the potential for liability (Chamorro & Tarulli, 1990).

Policy Issues

Public and private funding for home care is fragmented; payment for community-based services is limited; case management is uneven; funding for data collection and coordination is insufficient; and seamless health care systems are rudimentary, contributing to the difficulty in developing rational health policy for home care services (Goldberg & Frownfelter, 1990). Analysis of the use, role, purpose, effectiveness, and efficacy of both present and future technology used in home health care is increasingly important to the development of rational policy for patients, families, agencies, communities, private insurers, and local, state, and federal governments (Banta & Gelijins, 1994). Yet there is a paucity of reliable data concerning the home care use of many complex technologies. Much of this problem is attributable to the lack of available funding or reimbursement for data collection, analysis, and sophisticated research studies.

Assessment of technology and its use in the home is essential. This should include not only an overall assessment of the quality of care and patient outcomes for populations or communities of patients but also the quality of care and outcome for individual patients. As with other forms of health care, this requires attention to why, when, and how decisions are made about the appropriate use of medical technology in the home. Factors that place patients at risk in home care must be identified, especially for those who are dependent on complex technology.

Greater emphasis on electronic communication for home care is important for several reasons. It can improve overall productivity, reduce billing errors, and improve the charting of clinical and other data. Moreover, patient care data can be recorded at the point of care in the home rather than later in an office. Integration of the home care clinical record with the hospital's and nursing home's clinical data would create a way to monitor and oversee the quality, effectiveness, and cost of home care, as well as every aspect of health care (Gogola, 1995). Expanded and improved data and information systems are much needed in order to carefully craft policies on reimbursement, home care practice, quality and outcomes of care, access to care, family supports, and possible intermediate alternatives between care at home and in the hospital or nursing home (Arras & Dubler, 1994).

Severely disabled and technology-dependent persons can be cared for in their homes, but boundaries that have existed, and exist still, between hospitals, nursing homes, and community care make it difficult if not impossible to provide patients and families with integrated, coordinated, and seamless health care services. These boundaries must be reduced or eliminated if home and other segments of health care are to reach their full potential in improving patients' lives and possibly reducing the cost associated with institutional care (Bingley, 1993). Home care cannot be dissociated from other forms of care for those who are sick, disabled, and impaired; this is particularly evident for those who depend on technology for their very survival and well-being. Home care must become an integral part of health care systems, including disease prevention, health maintenance, ambulatory care of acute and chronic illnesses, hospitalization, rehabilitation, other institutional care, and home care. Integrated, seamless systems of health care, including home care, must be established and enhanced.

In summary, the United States has not yet determined how to manage or finance the growing older and younger populations of sick, disabled, and impaired persons who will receive technology-based home care. Yet the future expansion of such care seems certain, while its funding is uncertain. Unquestionably, there have been important achievements thus far, but there are many emerging issues associated with providing high-tech home care must be dealt with. These include the missing physician in home care (and long-term care generally); the challenges faced by nurses in providing and monitoring home care; the education and training of health care professionals; informing and supporting patients, families, and society; and balancing private and public responsibilities for financing and ensuring quality. Each of these issues must be dealt with and resolved in order for high-tech home care to grow successfully and without unduly burdensome increases in health care costs and expenditures.

REFERENCES

Abel, P. E. (1990). Ethics committees in home health agencies. *Public Health Nursing 7,* 256–259.

Alter, K. L. (1994). Tapping into new technology: Close links to patients at home. *Caring, 13*(2), 48–49.

Alemi, F., Stephens, R. C., Javalghi, R. G., Dyches, H., Butts, J., & Ghadiri, A. (1996). A randomized trial of a telecommunications network for pregnant women who use cocaine. *Medical Care, 34*(Suppl. 10), OS10–20.

Arno, P. S., Bonuck, K., & Padug, R. (1995). The economic impact of high-tech home care. In J. D. Arras (Ed.), *Bringing the hospital home: Ethical and social implications of high-tech home care* (pp. 220–234). Baltimore, MD: Johns Hopkins University Press.

Arras, J. D. (1994). The technological tether: An introduction to ethical and social issues in high-tech home care. *Hastings Center Report., 24*(5), S1–S2.

_____. (Ed.). (1995). *Bringing the hospital home: Ethical and social implications of high-tech home care.* Baltimore, MD: Johns Hopkins University Press.

Arras, J. D., & Dubler, N. N. (1994). Bringing the hospital home: Ethical and social implications of high-tech home care. *Hastings Center Report, 24*(5), S19–S28.

_____. (1995). Ethical and social implications of high-tech home care. In J. D. Arras (ed.), *Bringing the hospital home: Ethical and social implications of high-tech home care* (pp. 1–31). Baltimore, MD: Johns Hopkins University Press.

Banta, H. D., & Gelijins, A. C. (1994). The future and health care technology: Implications of a system for early identification. *World Health Statistics Quarterly, 47*(3–4), 140–148.

Bass, D. M., McClendon, M. J., Brennan, P. F., & McCarthy, C. (1998). The buffering effect of a computer support network on caregiver strain. *Journal of Aging and Health, 10*(1), 20–43.

Bernstein, L. H., Hankwitz, P. E., & Portnow, J. (1990). Home care of the elderly diabetic patient. *Clinical Geriatric Medicine, 6,* 943–957.

Bingley, J. D. (1993). Southport experience with domiciliary ventilation. *Paraplegia, 31*(3), 154–156.

Binstock, R. H. (1998). The financing and organization of long-term care. In L. C. Walker, E. H. Bradley, & T. Wetle (Eds.), *Public and private responsibilities in long-term care: Finding the balance* (pp. 1–22). Baltimore, MD: Johns Hopkins University Press.

Boling, P. A., & Keenan, J. M. (1992). Communication between nurses and physicians in home care. *Caring, 11*(5), 26–29.

Braunstein, M. L. (1993). The electronic patient records solution. *Caring, 12*(7) 30–33.

Brennan, P. F., Moore, S. M, & Smyth, K. (1995). The effect of a special computer network on care givers of persons with Alzheimer's disease. *Nursing Research, 33,* 166–172.

Brennan, P. F., & Ripich, S. (1994). Use of a home-care computer network by persons with AIDS. *International Journal of Technology Assessment in Health Care, 10*(2), 258–272.

Chamorro, T., & Tarulli, D. (1990). Strategies for risk management in cancer nursing. *Oncology Nursing Forum, 17,* 915–920.

Champlin, L. (1989). Home care goes "high-tech." *Geriatrics, 44*(7): 83–86.
deBlois, J. (1994). Changing the way we care for the dying *Health Programs, 75*(2), 48–49, 52.
Gogola, M. (1995). A joint hospital/vendor project brings CQI and point-of-care technology to home care. *Computers in Nursing, 13*(4), 143–150.
Goldberg, A. I. (1989). Home care for life-supported persons: The French system of quality control, technology assessment, and cost containment. *Public Health Reports, 104,* 329–335.
Goldberg, A. I., & Frownfelter, D. (1990). The ventilator-assisted individuals study. *Chest, 98*(2), 428–433.
Gustafson, D. H., Hawkins, R., Boberg, E., Pingree, S., Serlin, R. E., Graziano, F., & Chan, C. L. (1999). Impact of a patient-centered, computer-based health information/support system. *American Journal of Preventive Medicine, 16*(1), 1–9.
Haddad, A. M. (1992). Ethical problems in home healthcare. *Journal of Nursing Administration, 22*(3), 46–51.
Handy, C. M. (1989). Patient centered high-technology home care. *Holistic Nursing Practice, 3*(2), 46–53.
Hill, E. M. (1995). Perioperative management of patients with vascular disease. *AACN: Clinical Topics, 6,* 547–461.
Kastens, J. M. (1998). Integrated care management: aligning medical call centers and nurse triage services. *Nursing Economics, 16,* 320–322, 329.
Keenan, J. M., Hepburn, K. W., Ripsin, C. M., Webster, L. & Bland, C. J. (1992). A survey of Minnesota home care agencies perceptions of physician behaviors. *Family Medicine, 24*(2), 142–144.
Kenny, S., & Murray, B. (1993). New home-delivered training prospects for people with disabilities. *International Journal of Rehabilitation Research, 16*(3), 195–208.
Kwan, J. W., & Anderson, R. W. (1991). Pharmacists' knowledge of infusion devices. *American Journal of Hospital Pharmacy, 48*(10 Suppl. 1), S52–53.
Larkins, F. R., & Hellige, M. (1992). Adding high-tech home care services to your agency. *Caring, 11*(9), 18–22.
Lenane, J. C. (1994). High-tech cardiac home care. An emerging delivery system. *Life Watch, 13*(2), 28–31.
Liaschenko, J. (1994). The moral geography of home care. *Advances in Nursing Science, 17*(2), 16–26.
Lindberg, C. C. (1997). Implementation of in-home telemedicine in rural Kansas: Answering an elderly patient's needs. *Journal of the American Medical Informatics Association, 4*(1), 14–17.
Lindeman, C. A. (1992). Nursing and technology Moving into the 21st century. *Caring, 11*(9), 5, 7–10.

Marren, J. (1993). The real world experience: Death of homebound elderly persons: Staff views from the front lines. *Pride Institute Journal of Long Term Home Health Care, 12*(2), 42–45.

Meiners, M. R. (1996). The financing and organization of long-term care. In R. H. Binstock, L. E. Cluff, & O. von Mering (Eds.), *The future of long-term care: Social and policy issues* (pp. 191–214). Baltimore, MD: Johns Hopkins University Press.

Moller, G., Goldie, I. & Jonsson, E. (1992). Hospital care versus home care for rehabilitation after hip replacement. *International Journal of Technology Assessment in Health Care, 8*(1): 93–101.

Nathanson, M. D. (1996*). Home health care law manual.* Gaithersburg, MD: Aspen.

National Health Policy Forum. (1996). Medicare coverage for home health care: Reining in a benefit out of control (Issue Brief No. 694). Washington, DC: George Washington University.

O'Leary, S., Mann, C., & Perkash, I. (1991). Access to computers for older adults: Problems and solutions. *American Journal of Occupational Therapy, 45,* 636–642.

Parker, M. G., & Thorslund, M. (1991). The use of technical aids among community-based elderly. *American Journal of Occupational Therapy, 45,* 712–718.

Portnow, J. (1994). Assistive technology in home care. *Caring, 13*(9), 58–61.

Power, E. J. (1995). From the Congressional Office of Technology Assessment. *Journal of the American Medical Association, 27,* 4, 5.

Ripich, S., Moore, S. M., & Brennan, P. F. (1992). A new nurse medium: Computer networks for group intervention. *Journal of Psychosocial Nursing and Mental Health Services, 30*(7), 15–20.

Roe-Prior, P., Watts, R. J., & Burke, K. (1994). Critical care clinical nurse specialist in home health care: Survey results. *Clinical Nurse Specialist, 1,* 35–40.

Ross-Degnan, D., Soumerai, S. B., Avorn, J., Bohn, R. L., Bright, R., & Aledort, L. M. (1995). Hemophilia home treatment: Economic analysis and implications for health policy. *International Journal of Technology Assessment in Health Care, 11,* 327–344.

Sadock, J. M. (1995). Planning equipment acquisitions. *Journal of Health Resources Management, 13*(8), 16–21.

Sheldon, P., & Bender, M. (1994). High technology in home care: An overview of intravenous therapy. *Nursing Clinics of North America, 29,* 507–519.

Sherman, A. (1995). Critical care management of the heart failure patient in the home. *Critical Care Nursing Quarterly, 18*(1), 77–87.

Smith, C. E. (1994). A model of caregiving effectiveness for technology dependent adults residing at home. *Advances in Nursing Science, 17*(2), 27–40.

Smith, C. E., Geiffer, C. K., & Bieker, L. (1991). Technological dependency: A preliminary model and pilot of home total parenteral nutrition. *Journal of Community Health Nursing, 8,* 245–254.

Smith, C. E., Moushey, L., Ross, J. A., & Geiffer, C. K. (1993). Responsibilities and reactions of family caregivers of patients dependent on total parenteral nutrition at home. *Public Health, 10*(2), 122–128.

Weinstein, S. M. (1993). A coordinated approach to home infusion care. *Home Healthcare Nurse, 11*(1), 15–20.

White, M. C., & Smith, W. (1993). Infection control in home care agencies. *American Journal of Infection Control, 21*(3), 146–150.

Willging, P. (1995). The future of long-term care and the role of the medical director. *Clinical Geriatric Medicine, 11,* 531–545.

Williams, D. N. (1994). Reducing costs and hospital stay for pneumonia with home intravenous cefotaxime treatment: Results with a computerized ambulatory drug delivery system. *American Journal of Medicine, 97*(2A), 50–55.

Zwolski K. (1989). Nursing in a technical system. *Image—the Journal of Nursing Scholarship, 21*(4), 238–42.

CHAPTER 4

Families and Paid Workers: The Complexities of Home Care Roles

Baila Miller

The majority of home care workers in the United States are family members, other nonpaid sources of help, and older persons themselves. Even for persons with moderate or severe impairments, formal services, provided by paid workers, account for a relatively small share of the care provided to them (Grabbe, Demi, & Whittington, 1995; National Alliance for Caregiving and the American Association of Retired Persons, 1997). In a recent national survey, for example, older adults with functional impairments reported that they predominantly rely on informal sources of care, with less than 15% using formal home care (Norgard & Rodgers, 1997).

Yet the use of formal services is growing. During the past decade, expenditures for home health services have been one of the fastest growing components of the Medicare program (Gage, Stevenson, Korbin, & Aragon, 1998). Although there is no evidence that families use paid workers to substitute for informal care, as care needs increase, more older people and their families are likely to utilize formal care services to complement informal care (Ory, Hoffman, Yee, Tennstedt, & Shulz, 1999).

To date, there has been little research on the different home care roles of families and paid workers, and how they intersect. This chapter will outline a preliminary model for studying the role relationships between family and home care workers, illustrate these relationships with comments from families and workers obtained through field research, and examine policy implications. The chapter draws on the few qualitative studies in this area, including research in process (Biordi, Coehling, Miller, & Theis, 1993–1996), to give a grounded picture of possible role relationships between family members and home care workers. Given the range of stakeholders in the home care experiences (i.e., frail older relative, family member, professional health and social service caregivers, home aides, and general community caregivers), policy implications are complex.

SYMBOLIC MEANINGS OF HOME

Home is a broad concept. The major characteristic of home care, whether provided by family or paid workers, is that it is provided in private settings, behind closed doors (Fisher & Eustis, 1994). Home settings are characterized by the personal tastes and lifestyles of those who live there, a contrast to the institutionalized settings of hospitals and nursing homes.

The personalized setting of home can be both a strength and a source of tension in home care (Collopy, Dubler, & Zuckerman, 1990). As Robert Rubenstein (1990) noted:

> The term *home* is one of the richest symbols in Western culture.... Basic to the meanings of home are the various elements of control, security, family development, independence, comfort, protection, feelings, and the presence of people.... To keep a sick person at home, in essence, means that the person is not fully "sick." (p. 39)

Rubenstein added that when the home becomes a stage for the personal tasks of caregiving, paradoxes emerge. A major family goal of enabling a frail person to remain at home is to maintain independence and enhance quality of life. Yet this process often involves disturbing the usual domestic order of the home as a physical place, with changes in routine, organization of space, noise, odor, and so on. In addition, elderly home care recipients may be unwilling to accept increasing levels of dependence in the setting where they once functioned independently (Collopy et al., 1990). These disruptions in the symbolic and physical order of the home provide the context for understanding the relationship between family and home care provider.

INFORMALITY OF FORMAL CARE AND FORMALITY OF INFORMAL CARE

Gerontologists and sociologists often think in terms of dualities: home versus work; informal versus formal sources of help; public versus private spheres of influence and activity; instrumental versus emotional support. These intellectual concepts underlie our assumptions about the social world in which we live. Glazer (1990) argued that maintaining the archaic view of the privacy of the home and its separation from the core of social life inhibits our understanding of social relations. We thus lack the vocabulary to integrate and describe the personalizing emotional and instrumental aspects of work that has at its essence the goal of providing care for another human being (Aronson & Neysmith, 1996). We lack even a vocabulary to refer to the person needing care: patient, client, customer, consumer, or impaired older person. (This chapter will refer to the person in need as *client* or *older relative*.)

The concept of separation between public and private encourages policymakers to adopt the language of corporations in redefining human services according to business values and practices. One consequence of this is that the home, typically seen as a refuge and place of privacy, becomes reconstructed as a new health care marketplace that depends on self-care and women's domestic work (Glazer, 1990). At the same time, the instrumental task-oriented activities engaged in at home are given little value. The home can become a workshop (Glazer, 1990) in which professional, paraprofessional, and amateur family roles are blurred in the provision of tasks ranging from basic household activities (e.g., shopping) to high-technology medical service work. These dualities and lack of vocabulary are especially apparent as we examine the role of the family in home care, precisely because the use of home care involves the bridging of allegedly separate worlds.

Families and Paid Workers: The Complexities of Home Care Roles

The home setting encompasses the domains of family, client, and home care workers. The client, by virtue of need (i.e., functional or cognitive limitations) tends to be restricted to the home, with limited outside involvement. Although the client is the central focus (i.e., the person in need of care), family and workers typically relate to other systems of responsibility. Family caregivers are connected to broader support networks, other home-based and family activities, and work and community roles. Home care workers represent the formal support and the public arena. Their roles within the home care environment are complex and bounded not only by their relationship to the client, but also by their relationship to supervisors and their other social worlds. This combination of inward and outward perspectives is a theme permeating the catalog of family and paid-worker roles and relationships in home care.

MODEL OF FAMILY ROLES IN HOME CARE

Conceptualization of family roles in home care is in a state of research infancy. In view of the fragmented state of research in this area, and given the symbolic nature of family and home, I propose a heuristic model of factors that may contribute to variability in family role outcomes (see Figure 4.1). This model views family home care roles as embedded in a matrix of situational characteristics and family/personal characteristics. There are many areas of interdependency and feedback among these variables. In addition, outcome variables such as quality of home care and family and client physical and emotional well-being, could be added as a fourth dimension to this model.

This chapter, however, will focus on selected demand and contextual characteristics that may influence four primary family roles in home care: (1) *Provider role:* Family members alone provide care and are resistant to seek out other forms of home care; (2) *Task sharer role:* Family members share tasks with home care workers in complementary or substitutive ways; (3) *Broker role:* Family members take responsibility for locating and accessing sources of help; and (4) *Monitor role:* Family members become involved in the interpersonal relationships among family, older relatives, and home care workers.

We do not know yet if these roles are discrete or overlap in some type of continuum, nor do we know which roles are associated with what

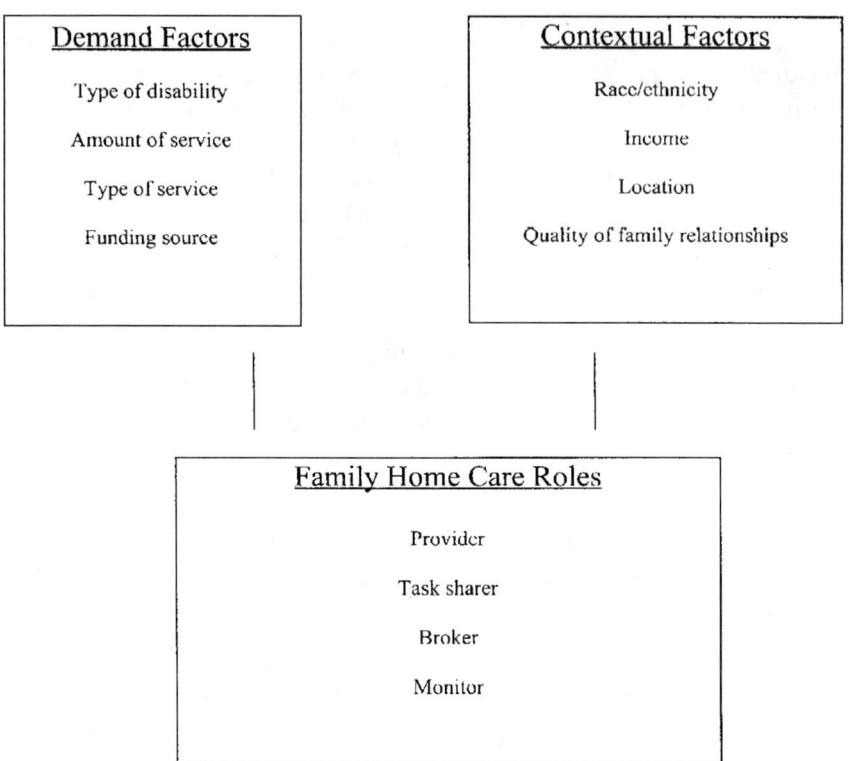

FIGURE 4.1 Model of family roles in home care.

types of demand characteristics. We also know little about how the effects of demand characteristics will be mediated by family and older relative resources such as income, ethnic and cultural factors, and degree of family burden or stress. Thus, this chapter is speculative, exploring how these dimensions may intersect with one another.

DEMAND CHARACTERISTICS

The type of client disability or need is a determining factor in the decision for home care. This decision is influenced by family and client resources, availability of services, and medical personnel. The relationship of disability to home care and the family and older person is interwoven with the funding source, type of home care worker, type of tasks and amount of service provided, and changes over time in client need. Thus, demand characteristics and their effect on the family can be separated in theory, but not in reality.

Type of disability also clearly influences the visibility and context of family roles. In situations of frailty with cognitively intact older relatives, the family may be relegated to a "backstage" role with the degree of stage management dependent on the quality of family relationships and the nature of other caregiving duties. For example, ". . . an 81-year-old married man requires a Hoyer lift to move from his bed to a wheelchair or from his chair to the toilet. He receives personal care and homemaking a few hours every day. His wife helps, but is too frail herself to either lift her husband or do extensive homemaking" (Fisher & Eustis, 1994, p. 293). Mobility and continence status overlay with other limitations in activities of daily living (ADLs) and instrumental activities of daily living (IADLs) to organize the type of tasks needed and provided. Bedridden clients require close personal care, meal preparation, and laundry, and are always almost totally dependent on aides and/or other caregivers. Similar tasks are needed for wheelchair-bound clients, especially assistance with bathing and toileting. For ambulatory alert clients, who may be suffering from diabetes, arthritis, or visual or hearing impairment, assistance with medication and household chores may be more prevalent (Feldman, Sapienza, & Kane, 1994).

Family members are more likely to be primary caregivers for persons with dementia and thus more heavily involved "on stage" in the home care decision and planning. Cognitively impaired older relatives in early to mid stages of dementia need supervision and companionship, rather than medically approved care. Home care workers are more likely to be paraprofessionals, who are expected to provide personal care and household help, and companionship. The definition of need for home care services for cognitively impaired persons straddles caregiver and older relative concerns. These services are often viewed as a respite for the caregiver as well as assistance for the older person. Eligibility requirements for many subsidized services for older persons rely on ADL limitations as screening mechanisms. Thus, formal home care workers are assigned only in more serious instances. Cognitively impaired clients present many difficulties for home care workers who have little understanding of or training in the implications of cognitive deficits and difficult behaviors that may accompany dementia. In addition, communication difficulties lead to a greater reliance on family communication than occurs with the functionally impaired but alert client.

The level and type of home care services can be described in terms of the education of the home care worker and related technology dimensions of "low-tech" versus "high-tech." Level of education and professionalism of home care workers varies. Professionally trained occupations that visit homes for specific tasks include occupational therapists, physical therapists, nurses, nutritionists, and social workers. These professionals tend to be responsible for assessment and certification of needs, development of care plans, and provision of direct medical, nursing, social, and other services. Much of their professionalism can be challenged in the home care setting by the potent threat of family and client authority to professional ideas of acceptable risk and appropriate conditions for care (Collopy et al., 1990).

Paraprofessionals include homemakers, home health aides, and chore workers who provide 70% to 80% of paid long-term home care. According to Crown (1994), the 1987–1989 Current Population Survey (CPS) reported that 93% of home care aides are women, with almost half (47.6%) widowed or divorced and about two thirds childless. Over 60% have at least a high school education, and half are between the ages of 45 and 64 years of age. These workers are typically paid an hourly wage of approximately $5.25 and work an average of 34.7 hours per week for approximately 42 weeks per year. Approximately 40% do not have health care benefits, while an additional 25% have employment-based health plans.

In an ongoing qualitative study of home and self-care, professionals were seen as shadowy figures in the respondents' stories. They were the persons who helped the older relative more with high technology than with treatments of body mechanics. Professional judgments were filtered through family patterns of care. As one family caregiver reported, "The doctor[s] didn't order physical therapy because they didn't think it would do [the client] any good. And it meant a lot of work for us, trying to keep her in good shape" (Biordi et al., 1993–1996).

Professionals and paraprofessional levels of care are not perfectly correlated with high- and low-tech home care situations. Low-tech home care is designed to help people maintain functional abilities or compensate for functional impairments. In low-tech care with alert mobile clients, the family members' involvement may be more on a symbolic level as a topic of conversation and/or observation by the worker than as a vivid presence. In care of the cognitively impaired client, the family may share care and supervision in a complementary or supplementary fashion. Low-tech home care may also be seen as respite for the caregiver or as supplementation of care that cannot be provided by family members.

High-technology care situations typically involve acute rather than chronic care (see chapter 3). Such care may involve infusion therapies or ventilator care. Family members often become willing or unwilling partners in high-tech care, under the pressure of swift hospital discharges that require them to learn rigorous routines such as sterilizing lines for parenteral feeding. Many older spouse caregivers resist or are unable to learn these techniques, or experience stress from carrying out such tasks and the life-or-death responsibility that may accompany them. Nurses are encouraged to teach home aides high-tech techniques if a family caregiver cannot be located or refuses to take on such tasks. As Glazer (1990) noted, "The highest level of care being done is in the home, but the people who are asked to do this are unskilled family members and/or minimum wage–level paid workers" (p. 492).

Funding sources and reimbursement systems create a different type of demand characteristic that can affect the course of home care more than clinical need of the care recipient under the current system (Cloonan, Phillips, Irvine, & Fisher, 1991; Schaffer, 1993). The types of services older persons are eligible for depends not only on their functional condition or diagnosis but also on their available insurance (Medicare, Medicaid, or private insurance) or ability to pay out-of-pocket. Many of the issues relating to access, accessibility, availability, and adequacy of care are the function of funding sources. (See chapter 1 for a fuller discussion of home care financing.) Medicare provides home health care services for acute care ordered by a physician upon discharge from a hospital. If a physician does not include "skilled" home care in the discharge plan, the prospective recipient may not receive Medicare coverage for home care services. Medicare does not pay for private duty nurses who are hired without physician's orders, homemaker services, or long-term custodial care. Many states currently are operating under Medicaid waiver plans, in which a variety of home care services are provided to older persons who are eligible for nursing home placement and meet the requirements of low-income and asset tests used by states to determine Medicaid eligibility. These programs are not restricted to medical services; depending on the specific circumstances of the client, they support adult day care, home chore services, respite care, custodial care, home meals and nutrition consultation, and durable medical equipment.

There are many ways that funding sources also influence family roles. One example is the restriction on amount of time a home care worker may be available. If only a 1-hour visit is permitted, home care workers are usually "too busy" to become involved with family members. Family members themselves may need to contribute more assistance. A second strain arises from the current fragmentation of home care services provided by public and third-party funding sources. Transportation, counseling, and light homemaking services may be provided by three different sources, each with its own set of rules and regulations. As one elderly client reported to her case manager, "I don't know who to tell what troubles to" (E. Stolarsky, personal communication, February 17, 1997).

CONTEXTUAL FACTORS

Little is known about the kinds of contextual factors that may mediate the emerging relationships between demand factors and the types of family roles. We may surmise from other research on families and long-term care that sociodemographics, gender, ethnicity and culture, geographical location, and history, quality, and type of family relationships will influence the shaping of family roles in home care. This chapter will not review the many studies in these areas, but rather focus on one example of how ethnicity and culture may mediate the relationship between demand characteristics and family roles. Ethnicity and culture may be especially important contextual factors because the home is a primary source of cultural transmission and enactment of values.

One way in which ethnicity and culture influence family roles is the misunderstanding in communication that may arise between members of different cultures compelled to work in close personal relationships. Randall-David (1989) and Sue (1990) set forth some generalizations regarding differences in communication styles that may create misunderstandings and discomfort. They suggest that African-Americans may rely on nonverbal communication for an assessment of true feelings, that conversational interruptions may be common and silence may indicate disagreement. Direct or personal questions, especially from a nonfamily member, may be perceived as harassment or an invasion of privacy. Among Asian-Americans, verbal styles tend to be nonaggressive, self-deprecating, indirect, and silent. A high value is placed on emotional restraint, with smiling used to mask uncomfortable feelings and to avoid conflict. It is considered inappropriate to be touched by a stranger, creating a problematic context for an Asian-American home care client or home care worker. Hispanics generally sit and stand closer to each other than Anglos and tend to touch people when speaking to them. Verbal styles are nonconfrontational and rarely offer encouraging communication to keep the conversation flowing.

The opportunities for cultural misunderstandings based on these verbal and nonverbal communication styles are obvious in the intimate informal-formal relationships that characterize home care. The extent to which the older client is able to be sensitive to cultural differences of the home care worker may be partly a function of the degree of discomfort associated with their functional and cognitive impairments. Anecdotal examples describe older persons and families making derogatory remarks about home care worker's habits (Eustis & Fischer, 1991). Conversely, workers may not understand the meaning or importance of certain rituals of care in the family (e.g., the importance of separate dairy and meat dishes in observant Jewish families) and disparage family or older client suggestions about appropriate ways of using a kitchen for meal preparation.

FAMILY ROLES IN HOME CARE

As explicated above, demand characteristics and contextual factors shape four roles that families play in relation to home care: provider role, task sharer role, broker role, and monitor role. There is little empirical evidence about the distribution and characteristics of these roles. Provider and task sharer roles emphasize the direct caregiving task assistance provided by family members to their frail older relative; the broker and monitoring roles reflect a more managerial stance by family members.

Provider Role

Although this chapter focuses on family and home care workers, the meaning that clients and their families attach to family caregiving without outside help is an important subtext in the story of home care. We have already noted that family members, especially spouses and adult daughters, are the majority of home care workers. For many families, home care services are simply unavailable, too expensive, appear to be of poor quality, or fail to mesh with the specific needs of the older person. Attitudes toward home care expressed by those who do not use such services provide an important perspective that underlies many feelings expressed about home care workers.

A major reason for nonuse of home care workers is refusal by the older relative to have help in the home. The central issue for many family members is not deciding that outside help is necessary, but convincing their elderly relative to accept it. This aspect can be especially problematic for adult child caregivers who are now caught in the need to assert control over the lives of their parents. Many older persons believe that they are managing, or that getting help means that they will lose their independence and start the slippery slope to a nursing home. In a Canadian study (Aronson, 1990), older respondents reported anxiety over the possibility that they would receive poor care from paid workers and anxiety about suffering diminishment because of loss of control of basic life circumstances. Although younger women in this study had a stronger sense of entitlement to service, they expressed concern about "grudgingly provided" public help.

Most persons and families are not socialized to place high monetary value on work performed in the home. Little societal consensus exists about the validity of spending one's savings on personal care needs. Current generations of older persons do place a high value on personal independence, and many perceive social stigmas to using personal care services. Thus, many older persons and families are reluctant to pay privately for home care, even if there are sufficient resources. Many also are reluctant to spend more than minimum wage to pay for sufficient hours of home and personal care. Even a minimum wage, however, can become expensive when many hours of care are needed and there is little third-party reimbursement.

A reluctance to claim entitlement to public services also reflects the strong belief that families are the proper context of care. Studies of family caregiving validate this point consistently (Horowitz, 1985; Stone, Cafferata, & Sangl, 1987). Families are also known to use fewer services than expected, even when such services are available in demonstration projects at little or no cost. In part, this behavior may stem from the family's reluctance to acknowledge need and inability to cope. It may also stem from the tendency of many family systems to exclude nonfamily sources of help. A few states are experimenting with paid family caregiving as one way of bridging this boundary issue, but such programs are limited (see Linsk, Keigher, Simon-Rusinowitz, & England, 1992). The idea of "home care worker as outsider" is vividly expressed by a bed-ridden older African-American woman, who is cared for by her niece as a paid family caregiver:

> Well it's like a private thing that I would be more comfortable with her than an outsider. And I'm taken care of every way. I have just about everything I need. I eat my meals on time; I get baths every day, change of linen, clothes. It's like, basically, it's real hard for another person cause I know, she's from outside. An outsider would come in and maybe they would do it and maybe they wouldn't or whatever. But it's just comfortable with her. So I feel very good about it. (Biordi et al., 1993–1996)

As this quotation indicates, the expectation that family members are the most appropriate providers of care is powerful.

Task Sharer Role

The policy perspective of containing public expenditures for home care drives much of the research on the relationship between formal and informal sources of help. A central issue is whether the availability of public funding for services will cause a substitution of formal care for informal care, thereby "unnecessarily" inflating government costs. Studies consistently show that families do not stop providing care when home care services are used (Miller & McFall, 1991; Noelker & Bass, 1989). Supplementary and complementary patterns of help are the norm, not substitution. For certain kinds of tasks (e.g., transportation), there is a greater likelihood of both informal and formal helpers providing assistance, albeit at different times. For other tasks, especially personal care such as bathing, a home care worker may be called in to provide help when the caregiver, often an elderly frail spouse, is no longer able to carry out the task. Many home care workers provide extra help (e.g., doing errands). For example, one home care worker described, "I've taken [the client] to weddings and to anniversaries and to funerals. She pays for the gas, but I don't let her pay me for the hours I spend with her" (Eustis & Fischer, 1991, p. 450).

An ongoing tension in home care is the diffuse job responsibilities that accompany homemaking and chore service activities and idiosyncratic individual parameters of the work role. There may be a conflict between individual, nonstandardized knowledge of the family caregiver versus the standardized solutions of the home care professional. "We do what the professionals tell us . . . but, if he wears the other prosthesis all day like she wants him to, then he has to have the other footrest on the wheelchair and then he can't get into the bathroom or anything, our house is so small" (Hasselkus, 1988, p. 689). In other instances, family caregivers may use the presence of home care professionals to learn better ways of managing. "This morning, I had [the nurse] show me how she [uses the Hoyer lift]. I think her way is easier" (Hasselkus, 1988, p. 689).

Even nonprofessional home care workers frequently provide an educational experience for family caregivers, acting as "bumble bees" who pass along information about how other families manage. Most families have little opportunity to learn about improving care management. Hughes (1989) found that when a home team intervention emphasized the importance of caregiver training, along with supervision and monitoring of patient, family members became more confident and secure in their caregiving roles.

When family members share tasks, they need to find ways to separate their contributions from home care workers. One approach is to define their unique contribution in terms of the emotional and affiliative ties between the older relative and family caregivers. In other words, family members emphasize that professional home care workers couldn't provide love. As one caregiver noted, "I know nurses are wonderful and can do a lot of things I can't stomach to do. Right now, I don't need to do a lot of things that I can't stomach, so, the love that I can give her in what I do is premium. It's like the added value. It's that extra I can put into her life" (Biordi et al., 1993–1996).

Normalization of caregiving responsibilities is another way of distinguishing family caregiving activities from home care workers. Normal household activities are emphasized as noncaregiving activities compared to special tasks occasioned by the older relative's frailty or impairment. Those family caregivers who view care as a family obligation and see service use as an admission of failure to manage by themselves can avoid guilty feelings by defining unique family care roles for themselves.

Broker Role

The range of activities involved in arranging for home care creates a challenge to the family member who experiences a need for "some additional help around the house" with their impaired relative. Caregivers, especially adult children with greater economic resources, spend much of their time arranging for services. The home care service world is a crazy quilt of fragmented services. Family members must maneuver through different sources of service provision, each with its own eligibility and funding patterns. Organizing and coordinating different sources of different services becomes a major task.

A large degree of uncertainty overlays the broker role. This uncertainty and vulnerability are expressed by an adult daughter of an ailing mother:

> This one person that I've hired to help me is a lovely person, very nice, very nice. But I don't know how long she'll be with us, because you never know what someone else's life will be. You're really dealing from weakness, so you just have to kind of do what you can to please them. You tend to bend over backwards for the help because it's so hard to find this kind of help and I'm very particular. I'm not a person that's just going to call an agency and say "Send somebody over." (Abel, 1991, p. 141)

Issues of family autonomy and control are involved in many of the decisions made as part of the broker role. Families applying to publicly supported service agencies are faced with eligibility requirements and loss of control over the amount and mix of services and the choice of worker. Agencies that provide professional assessment and sliding-scale fees can provide a valuable resource for families who are comfortable accepting professional judgment in lieu of family beliefs about appropriate types of care. Families who hire paid workers privately are faced with locating sources of help, filing tax forms, dealing with no-shows, and so on, but maintain fuller control over the process. Because the majority of individuals who can afford to make private arrangements for home care workers, relying on word of mouth, the need for family control appears to be important.

Monitor Role

The role of monitoring home care services is the most complex and problematic for family members, older relatives, home care workers, and organizations that employ and provide home care workers for others. The ambiguity of the relationships among home care worker and older person and family members is due in part to the informality of formal relationships. The personal, private, and intrusive nature of care by the home care worker creates a unique working environment. The quality of interpersonal relationships and ability to engender a sense of trust become as important as task-related skills. Eustis and Fisher (1991) reported that almost two thirds of clients and half of workers used noncontractual terms such as *friend* or *like family* in defining these relationships. (See also Karner, 1998, for an elaboration of home care workers as fictive kin.)

Although home care users value the health care skills of workers, some would prefer adequate care from a worker with whom they had a good relationship than excellent care given by an unpleasant worker. The importance of trust is evidenced by stories of mistrust in which families accuse workers of theft or of cheating on hours, and also by stories of extensive trust, in which workers pay bills for clients and keep track of their own hours (Eustis & Fisher, 1991).

Most client complaints are not about job performance, but about interpersonal dynamics and lack of compatibility between client and worker. This element of interpersonal relationship is also important to formal providers of home care. Home care workers cite good relationships with clients as one of the most valued components of their work.

A study of worker-client interaction by Eustis and Fischer (1991) identified four patterns of family-worker relationships that encompass the tensions and ambiguity between informal and formal relationships in family-relative-worker roles: personal, formal, asymmetrical, and collegial. Little is known about what characteristics of the home care worker or older person or family contribute to a specific type of relationship or what types of relationship are associated with higher quality of care. Clarifications and modifications of the four patterns can be discerned in comments made by family caregivers and home care workers in a variety of studies.

Personal

Familiar and friendlike behavior characterizes the interaction. Personal problems of both workers and family or older relative are shared in mutual socializing and confiding interactions. This pattern may be more prevalent in rural areas and in long-term relationships whether rural, urban, or suburban. Yet, as one home care worker suggests, such personal or collegial relationships can give rise to complications:

> I had been thinking about Joe [the client] as a friend and I am still trying to sort my thoughts out about this—because there is a fine line here. I have worked really hard to relate to him and get to know him. I thought we had gotten to be friends.... He told me things about himself and his family. And then it was really hard when he barked at me." (Eustis & Fisher, 1991, p. 452)

Formal

Lack of familiar and friend-like behavior, with little confiding or socializing. This pattern may be more typical in urban areas in which home care workers are assigned by formal organizations and carefully monitored by funding sources. Even in formal relationships, however, the skills that are appreciated are apt to be relationship-based, rather than technical. Workers who are mindful of the loss of independence experienced by the older relative are especially appreciated. An adult daughter-caregiver described an ideal home care worker:

> Joan has these extra skills of observation and supervision which she does subtly that my mother thinks she's not doing anything. That's the biggest gift of all. I don't know if you can train somebody to do that, and do it as well as this woman does it. She just has a natural gift of it, to always make my mother feel as though she's making every decision, doing everything on her own, when really Joan is right there helping." (Abel, 1991, p. 452)

Asymmetrical

Imbalance in reciprocity, where the client may think of the relationship as familial, but little mutual confiding takes place. Clients are more likely to share their personal problems with workers than workers are to confide in their clients. Many workers make comments about not wanting to burden their clients with their problems. They believe that clients had enough troubles of their own to take care of and may share their concerns selectively to cheer up or entertain a client (Eustis & Fischer, 1991).

One adult daughter-caregiver hints at an asymmetrical relationship when her regular nurses are unable to visit:

I've got a rapport with these two. I was actually sort of frantic because a couple of others who've come in at different times, they just weren't . . . they just didn't seem to have the same rapport. It's very difficult to get into conversation with them, apart from a purely medical thing about Mum. (Opie, 1992, p. 166)

Yet another type of asymmetrical relationship is cited by a home care worker caring for a person with dementia:

What I like most is giving her [the client] love and warmth and treating her like a human being. The love I give her keeps her going. Here, I'm helping someone and I know I'm appreciated. She reaches out and grabs my hand, kisses my cheek and says, "I love you." And then says nothing for the next six months. Those times when she can show her love are worth everything. (Feldman et al., 1994, p. 19).

Collegial

There is recognition of mutuality, but in the context of a working professional relationship. Few examples of this form of relationship appear in the literature.

Anecdotal evidence from family caregivers provides glimpses of negative reactions to home care, but the prevalence of these is not well documented. Areas of distrust can be based on cultural and educational differences between home care workers and family. Some family members have difficulties establishing boundaries to the service provider and may have unrealistic expectations. "It wouldn't hurt if they would come over and relieve me so I could have a day off" (Biordi et al., 1993–1996) or "It would be nice to have them around for the holidays" (Fisher & Eustis, 1994, p. 300). Home care workers also have complaints about families. "Families are the hard thing to work with. One usually takes care of the whole thing and the others tell you what to do" (Fisher & Eustis, 1994, p. 300). Interestingly, even though positive reactions appear to be more common than negative, persons who do not receive home care services are more likely to repeat negative stories they have heard than positive ones (Miller & Stull, 1999).

POLICY IMPLICATIONS

The policy context for the relationships among clients, families, and paid workers in home care lies in the long-term care arena. Long-term care policy is often described as decentralized, categorical, and limited, relying heavily on implementation of federal initiatives through state authority and discretion (Benjamin, 1992). Most federal and state policies regarding home care are based on the premise of cost containment and the assumption that families are the first line of defense in meeting the needs of family members. The goal is ensuring that publicly funded formal care does not replace the informal care provided by the family. Formal surrogates are perceived as necessary only when families are unavailable or unable to carry out their responsibilities (Hendricks & Rosenthal, 1993). Promoting the well-being of caregivers has not been a policy goal, and the rights of caregivers to public support have not been recognized within long-term care policies. Policies have concentrated on the dependent older person, not the interconnections between the older person and those who provide care (Osterbusch, Keigher, Miller, & Linsk, 1987). These value constraints and what is known about the complexity of family roles in home care suggests three primary policy issues related to family roles.

The first issue concerns how to take family needs into account in determining eligibility for service and details of care plans. The notion of what constitutes a family is in great flux. The boundaries of traditional ideas of the intergenerational family based on a nuclear model have been blurred, almost beyond recognition. We now have gay parents, grandparent-headed households, step families, dual-earner couples, and commuter marriages instead of the idealized nuclear families. In addition to discretionary families and conventional families, there are growing numbers of "everyday families" of fictive kin of peers, friends, and neighbors. These relationships share typical characteristics of a family such as affection and solidarity, regular interaction, and sense of obligation to provide care (Karner, 1998; Sussman, 1985).

The definition of who is a family member has policy relevance. For example, to be eligible for the Federal Dependent Care Tax Credit, the taxpayer must not only supply over 50% of the dependent's economic support but also spend at least 8 hours a day in the household (Hooyman

& Gonyea, 1995). Thus, adult children or other relatives or friends who live near a dependent parent cannot claim the tax credit even if they provide extensive economic or instrumental support.

A second issue is the potential usefulness of paying family caregivers. Typically, family caregivers, most of whom are women, are economically penalized by their roles as unpaid caregivers in the home. Compensation for provision of care needs to be oriented toward the caregivers' well-being, in addition to decreasing costs through avoiding nursing home placement (Hooyman and Gonyea, 1995). Stone & Keigher (1994) suggest that financial supports for caregivers should (1) be sufficient to achieve and maintain a decent standard of living, (2) be fairly distributed among caregivers who meet a certain standard of need, and (3) be compatible with caregivers' other family and social needs. At the same time, there must be recognition that formal home care will continue to be needed to provide caregiver relief.

A third issue concerns the rigidity of defining reimbursement policies for home care solely in terms of concrete tasks. Should some time for attending to the interpersonal and relationship needs of older clients and families be included? As Eustis, Kane, and Fisher (1993) ask, "As a matter of public policy, is the client "owed" a good relationship with a publicly paid caregiver? Is the worker owed time to attend to her client's emotional needs?" (p. 71). A clear message from the few studies on families, clients, and home care workers is the value that they place on the informality of the formal relationships and the importance of trust-building skills. Current funding standards focus on a task approach, detailing exactly what tasks and time should be spent on each client, rather than understanding the balance between competence and good relationship. Interpersonal needs must be justified under restrictive mental health funding criteria, with counseling then provided as a separate "task."

Rigid emphasis on task provision only may compromise the value of maintaining the older person in the community. The importance of developing working partnerships among family members, older relative, and home care personnel is an important theme in the practice literature (see Feldman, 1994). Yet promoting such partnerships is a substantial challenge because of the realities of cost containment and the difficulties of distinguishing between an impaired client's need for socializing from his or her more general needs for friendship.

Perhaps, the most important home care policy issue is the general lack of access to paid home care. Fisher and Eustis (1994) aptly commented:

"Care at home is expensive—in time and/or money. In this country, most individuals with long-term care needs and most family caregivers cannot afford much or any paid home care" (p. 308). Families and individuals with moderate incomes are often not eligible for the publicly funded programs based on financial need (i.e., Medicaid waiver programs). Individuals with functional disabilities and chronic conditions are rarely eligible for Medicare reimbursement, which requires recipients to be homebound and in need of intermittent services under medical direction. Moreover, the growing emphasis on managed care threatens even this limited provision of care. According to one study, the average Medicare patient enrolled in a health maintenance organization received about two thirds as many home health care visits as a Medicare patient with traditional fee-for-service coverage (Schlenker, Shaughnessy, Hittle, 1995). Thus, the challenge of integrating family roles in home care policy and expanding affordable home care continues.

REFERENCES

Abel, E. (1991). *Who cares for the elderly? Public policy and the experiences of adult daughters.* Philadelphia: Temple University Press.

Aronson, J. (1990). Women's perspectives on informal care of the elderly: Public ideology and personal experience of giving and receiving care. *Ageing and Society, 10,* 61–84.

Aronson, J., & Neysmith, S. (1996). You're not just in there to do the work: Depersonalizing policies and the exploitation of home care worker's labor. *Gender and Society, 19,* 59–77.

Benjamin, A. J. (1992). An overview of in-home health and supportive services for older persons. In M. G. Ory & A. P. Duncker (Eds.), *In-home care for older people* (pp. 9–52). Newbury Park, CA: Sage.

Biordi, D., Coehling, H., Miller, B., & Theis, S. (1993–1996). In-home care and respite care as self care (National Institute for Nursing Research, RO1-NRO-3532).

Cloonan, P. A., Phillips, E. K., Irvine, A., & Fisher, M. E. (1991). Study of patients receiving no billed nursing care. *Home Health Care Services Quarterly, 12*(1), 37–45.

Collopy, B., Dubler, N., & Zuckerman, C. (1990). The ethics of home care: Autonomy and accommodation. *Hastings Center Report* (March/April), 1–16.

Crown, W. H. (1994). A national profile of home care, nursing home, and hospital aides. *Generations, 18*(3), 29–33.

Eustis, N. N., & Fischer, L. R. (1991). Relationships between home care clients and their workers: Implications for quality of care. *Gerontologist, 31,* 447–456.

Eustis, N. N., Kane, R. A., & Fisher, L. R. (1993). Home care quality and the home care worker: Beyond quality assurance as usual. *Gerontologist, 33,* 64–73.

Feldman, P. H. (Ed.). (1994). Frontline workers in long-term care. *Generations, 18* (3).

Feldman, P. H., Sapienza, A. M., & Kane, N. M. (1994). On the home front: The job of the home aide. *Generations, 18*(3), 16–19.

Fischer, L. R., & Eustis, N. N. (1994). Care at home: Family caregivers and home care workers. In E. Kahana, D. E. Biegel, & M. L. Wykle (Eds.), *Family caregiving across the lifespan* (pp. 287–311). Thousand Oaks, CA: Sage.

Gage, B., Stevenson, D., Korbin, L., & Aragon, C. (1998). Medicare home health: An update. *Public Policy and Aging Report, 9*(3), 12–15.

Glazer, N. (1990). The home as workshop: Women as amateur nurses and medical care providers. *Gender and Society, 4,* 479–499.

Grabbe, L., Demi, A. S., & Whittington, F. (1995). Functional status and the use of formal home care in the year before death. *Journal of Aging and Health, 7,* 339–364.

Hasselkuss, B. R. (1988). Meaning in family caregiving: Perspectives on caregiver/professional relationships. *Gerontologist, 28,* 686–691.

Hendricks, J., & Rosenthal, C. J. (Eds.). (1993). *The remainder of their days: Domestic policy and older families in the United States and Canada.* New York: Garland.

Hooyman, N. R., & Gonyea, J. (1995). *Feminist perspectives on family care.* Thousand Oaks, CA: Sage.

Horowitz, A. (1985). Family caregiving to the frail elderly. *Annual Review of Gerontology and Geriatrics, 5,* 194–246.

Hughes, S. (1989). Home and community care of the elderly: System resources and constraints. In J. A. Barondness, E. D. Rogers, & K. N. Lohr (Eds.), *Care of the elderly patient: Policy issues and research opportunities* (pp. 55–610). Washington, DC: National Academy Press.

Karner, T. X. (1998). Professional Caring: Homecare workers as fictive kin. *Journal of Aging Studies, 12*(1), 69–82.

Linsk, N., Keigher, S., Simon-Rusinowitz, L., & England, S. (1992). *Wages for caring: Compensating family care of the elderly.* New York: Praeger.

Miller, B., Campbell, R. T., Davis, L., Furner, S., Giachello, A., Prohaska, T., Kaufman, J. E., Li, M., & Perez, C. (1996). Minority use of community long-term care services: A comparative analysis. *Journal of Gerontology: Social Sciences, 51B,* S70–S81.

Miller, B., & McFall, S. (1991). The effect of caregiver burden on change in formal task support of frail older persons. *Journal of Health and Social Behavior, 32,* 165–179.

Miller, B., McFall, S., & Campbell, R. T. (1994). Changes in sources of community long-term care among African-Americans and white frail older persons. *Journal of Gerontology: Social Sciences, 49,* S14–S24.

Miller, B., & Stull, D. (1999). Perceptions of community services by African-American and White older persons. In M. Wykle & A. Ford (Eds.), *Serving minority elders in the 21st century* (pp. 267–286). New York: Springer.

National Alliance for Caregiving and the American Association of Retired Persons. (1997). *Family caregiving in the U.S.: Findings from a national survey* (final report). Bethesda, MD: National Alliance for Caregiving.

Noelker, L. S., & Bass, D. M. (1989). Home care for elderly persons: Linkages between formal and informal caregivers. *Journal of Gerontology: Social Sciences, 44,* S63–S70.

Norgard, T. M., & Rodgers, W. L. (1997) Patterns of in-home care among elderly black and white Americans [Special issue]. *Journals of Gerontology: Series B, 52B,* 93–101.

Opie, A. (1992). *There's nobody there: Community care of confused older people.* Philadelphia: University of Pennsylvania Press.

Ory, M. G., Hoffman, R. R., III, R. R., Yee, J. L., Tennstedt, S., & Schulz, R. (1999). Prevalence and impact of caregiving: A detailed comparison between dementia and nondementia caregivers. *Gerontologist, 39,* 177–185.

Osterbusch, S., Keigher, S., Miller, B., & Linsk, N. (1987). Community care policies and gender justice. *International Journal of Health Services, 17,* 217–232.

Randall-David, E. (1989). *Strategies for working with culturally diverse communities and clients.* Bethesda, MD: Association for Care of Children's Health.

Rubenstein, R. L. (1990). Culture and disorder in the home care experience: The home as sickroom. In J. F. Gubrium & A. Sankar (Eds.), *The home care experience: Ethnography and policy* (pp. 37–58). Newbury Park, CA: Sage.

Schaffer, C. L. (1993). Regulator structure of home health care in the United States. *Journal of Cross-cultural Gerontology, 8,* 407–416.

Schlenker, R. E., Shaughnessy, P. W., & Hittle, D. F. (1995). Patient-level cost of home health care under capitated and fee-for-service payment. *Inquiry, 32,* 252–270.

Stone, R., Cafferata, G., & Sangl, J. (1987). Caregivers of the frail elderly: A national profile. *Gerontologist, 27,* 616–626.

Stone, R., & Keigher, S. (1994). Toward an equitable universal caregivers policy: The potential of financial supports for family caregivers. *Aging and Social Policy, 6,* 57–76.

Sue, D. (1990). *Counseling the culturally different: Theory and practice.* New York: Wiley.
Sussman, M. B. (1985). The family life of old people. In R. H. Binstock & E. Shanas (Eds.), *Handbook of aging and the social sciences* (2nd ed., pp. 415–449). New York: Van Nostrand Reinhold.

CHAPTER 5

Hospice: End-of-Life Care at Home

Patrice C. Moore
Robert H. McCollough

As indicated in a 1997 report from the Institute of Medicine, National Academy of Sciences (Field & Cassel, 1997), much attention is being given to improving care at the end of life in hospitals, nursing homes, and day care centers, and in homes where there are terminally ill patients. Emphasis has been given to (1) increasing awareness of people with advanced and potentially fatal illnesses of the care they need and that should be available to them; (2) increasing the knowledge, awareness, and effectiveness of nurses, physicians, and others responsible for the care of terminally ill persons; (3) developing policies and strategies to improve the measuring, financing, regulation, and coordination of care of the terminally ill; (4) expanding the research and analyses required to better understand the needs and care of those with serious, disabling, advanced, and potentially fatal illnesses; and (5) developing a better personal and public understanding of the realities of the process of dying and of death.

Since major scientific and technologic advances in medicine and surgery began to take place following World War II, public and personal attention has progressively looked to physicians and medical institutions to provide "miraculous" treatments and cures for disease. Indeed, such advances have materially reduced or eliminated the ravages of many disastrous acute and chronic illnesses. Yet, even though medical care may prolong life, it cannot prevent death and dying. So there is a need to provide supportive and compassionate care for those who no longer can be cured or have their lives prolonged by medical or surgical treatments.

Hospice services, which are primarily provided in the home, directly address this need. They also carry out the missions outlined by the report from the Institute of Medicine. The goals of hospice care are to provide a good quality of life for the dying person and to help the patient and family (or caregiver) deal with approaching death, emphasizing palliative care of the patient, rather than curing the patient's disease or extending life.

Although hospice care usually takes place in the home of a dying person, it also can be provided in other residential and institutional settings. As described by the National Hospice Organization (Connor, 1998), hospice is

> ...a coordinated program providing palliative care to terminally ill patients and supportive services to patients, their families, and significant others 24 hours a day, seven days a week. Comprehensive/case managed services based on physical, social, spiritual, and emotional needs are provided during the last stages of illness, during the dying process, and during bereavement by a medically directed interdisciplinary team consisting of patients/families, health care professionals and volunteers. Professional management and continuity of care is maintained across multiple settings including homes, hospitals, long term care and residential settings. (pp. 3–4)

There is a general lack of awareness of hospices and the purposes of the palliative care they provide. To palliate is to lessen the pain or severity of disease, without curing. This can be accomplished in many different ways. Death, of course, is the ultimate palliative event. Prior to death there are many who experience the violence of diseases that may be acute, chronic and progressive, chronic and progressive with remittances, or terminal. Palliative care for such persons can relieve pain, anxiety, depression, isolation, and other manifestations of disease that can ravage both patients who are terminally ill and their families. Yet it often appears that physicians are not familiar with hospice as an organized way to provide palliation and supportive care for dying patients and their families.

This chapter provides an overview of hospices and the patients they serve, mostly through care in the home. First, it traces the development of hospice in the United States, which was substantially spurred by federal funding. Second, it presents a picture of who is eligible for hospice care and insurance benefits. Third, it discusses the settings for hospice care and the characteristics of hospice patients. Fourth, it describes hospice services in detail. Finally, it sets forth some ongoing challenges involving hospice care.

THE DEVELOPMENT OF HOSPICE IN THE UNITED STATES

Although the concept of hospice dates to 361 A.D. (Stoddard, 1992), the growth of the modern hospice movement is widely accepted to be the result of the efforts of Dame Cicely Saunders. In 1967 she established St. Christopher's Hospice in Sydenham, outside London. The seeds for development of hospice in the United States were planted in 1965 when Florence Wald, then the dean of the Yale School of Nursing, invited Dame Saunders to become a visiting faculty member. Subsequently, Wald and Edward F. Dobhal, Jr., clinical professor of pastoral care at Yale Divinity School, reviewed the model of St. Christopher's Hospice while on sabbatical in London during the late 1960s. In 1971 Wald, Dobhal, and others were instrumental in opening the Connecticut Hospice in New Haven, marking the first formal hospice program in the United States (Stoddard, 1992).

The hospice movement that began in the early 1970s in the United States changed the way care was provided to dying people and altered the expectations dying people and their loved ones had of the health care system. In the early days of hospice in America, grassroots groups, religious groups, and health care providers intent on providing an alternative to traditional health care gathered together with like-minded people committed to offering more humane care for individuals facing the end of their life.

The model of hospice as it was defined in England became broader in the United States, with greater emphasis on care in home settings. Instead of providing hospice care exclusively under one roof in a facility, care was brought to the patient rather than having the patient move into a facility.

Prior to any state or federal regulations, American hospices were essentially composed of volunteer groups offering mostly nursing and supportive assistance, doing any number of tasks the patient and family requested. The most important of these hospice activities were (as they are today) the provision of emotional support for the family or loved ones and managing the patient's pain, discomforts, and fears.

In the decade that followed the introduction of hospice in the United States, it gradually emerged on the national public policy agenda, substantially increasing care options for terminally ill patients. In 1974, just 3 years after it was formed, the Connecticut Hospice received a grant from the National Cancer Institute to develop a national demonstration center for home care for the terminally ill and their families. National recognition and legitimization of the hospice movement grew steadily in the years that followed. In 1978 a U.S. Department of Health, Education, and Welfare task force reported that "the hospice movement as a concept for the care of the terminally ill and their families is a viable concept and one which holds out a means of providing more humane care for Americans dying of terminal illness while possibly reducing costs. As such, it is the proper subject of federal support" (American Hospice Association, 1999). In 1979 the Health Care Financing Administration (HCFA) funded demonstration programs at 26 hospices across the United States to assess the cost effectiveness of hospice care and to identify the services that hospice should provide.

The first publicly funded hospice benefit was established by the Tax Equity and Fiscal Responsibility Act of 1982, which made it available to participants in Part A of the federal Medicare health insurance program (99% of Americans age 65 and older, persons receiving federal disability insurance, and individuals with end-stage renal disease). This Medicare hospice benefit (MHB), authorized on a temporary basis through 1986, was limited by caps on both overall annual aggregate per-patient payments and inpatient hospital utilization (at 20% of total patient "at home" days). To implement these limits, HCFA created a prospective payment system for the MHB, which is a flat daily rate based on one of four levels of care—routine care, continuous care, respite care, and general inpatient care—regardless of the extent of care provided.

Congress made the MHB permanent in 1986, and reimbursement rates were increased by 10%. In addition, states were allowed the option of including hospice as a covered benefit under Medicaid, the federal-state health insurance program for the poor. In 1989 Congress provided an additional rate increase for the MHB and tied future increases to the annual rate of inflation in hospital costs. A year later the existing 210-day lifetime benefit limitation under the MHB was removed.

In 1991 hospice care was also authorized in military hospitals under the Civilian Health and Medical Program of the Uniformed Services (CHAMPUS) in the National Defense Authorization Act. A commission on health care for veterans also released a report that year, recommending inclusion of hospice care in the veteran's benefit package (Commission on the Future Structure of Veterans' Health Care, 1991). The CHAMPUS hospice benefit was finally implemented in June 1995.

The establishment of the MHB, more than any other social, political, or biomedical event since the founding of the hospice movement in Great Britain, has had a profound effect on how dying is managed in the United States (Billings, 1998). It markedly changed the way that care is provided at the end of life by transforming hospice from a predominantly volunteer-staffed activity on the fringes of organized medicine, into a professional activity carried out within the mainstream of the American health care system. An indication of this change is that from 1986 (when the MHB was permanently established) to 1996, Medicare payments of hospice benefits increased by 2,500%, from just $77 million to $2 billion, with most of this growth attributable to increases in the number of beneficiaries receiving hospice care (Health Care Financing Administration, 1998).

In 1982, when an MHB was first created, there were only about 500 hospices nationwide, with few of them offering a full range of hospice services. One third were freestanding programs; the rest were attached to hospitals and home health agencies. None were financially viable. They all functioned through the volunteer and financial generosity of their communities and/or their parent health care organizations. Services were limited to mostly white, middle-class people with diagnosed cancer who also had informal caregiving support from family, other kin, or friends (Mahoney, 1998).

By 1997 there were about 3,100 operational or planned hospice programs in the United States (including the District of Columbia and Puerto Rico), providing care for approximately 495,000 patients annually.

Approximately 65% of hospices were not-for-profit, 16% were for-profit, 4% were government organizations (e.g., Department of Veterans Affairs), and 15% were "other" or unidentified (Mahoney, 1988).

About 10% of the agencies providing hospice care in 1996 were in the Northeast region, 35% in the Midwest, 40% in the South, and 16% were in the West. Sixty-three of the agencies were located in a metropolitan statistical area (Advance Data, 1998a).

ELIGIBILITY AND BENEFITS

To be eligible for the MHB, patients admitted for hospice care must be referred by a physician and terminally ill, with a prognosis of dying within 6 months, and prepared to accept supportive and palliative care only. It must have been determined by the physician that no further "curative" medical care is planned or likely to be effective (U.S. Codes of Federal Regulations, 1993). The 6-month requirement does not necessarily mean that patients who survive this period must be dropped from hospice programs (although there are occasions when patients who become stable or are in a remission are discharged because they no longer meet the criteria of being terminally ill with 6 months to live). The patient who is steadily declining may remain in the hospice program if both the referring physician and the medical director of the hospice agree that the individual's condition continues to be terminal, with 6 months to live. With this type of status review, two 90–day benefit periods (U.S. Code of Federal Regulations, 1993) and, subsequently, an unlimited number of 60–day periods (Palmetto Government Benefit Administrators, 1997) are available.

For patients who meet MHB eligibility criteria, four levels of care are reimbursable. *Level 1,* the most common, is hospice care of the terminally ill living at home or in other residential settings such as an assisted living facility, a hospice residence (hospice house), or a nursing home. This benefit covers the services of physician, nurse, social worker, chaplain, and volunteer, as well as bereavement care for the family. Professional team visits are scheduled according to patient and family need, and nursing services are available, as needed, 24 hours a day, 7 days a week. Also covered are medical equipment and supplies and drugs that relieve symptoms such as pain. For some patients, the MHB drug benefit (which has a very small co-insurance payment) is the deciding factor in a decision to enter a hospice program. The expense of opioids, for example, can be several hundred dollars a week.

The *Level 2* benefit covers continuous care. Private duty care is provided 24 hours a day for short periods in times of crisis, to manage the patient at home. *Level 3* covers respite care in a hospital or nursing home facility for up to 5 days, per stay, providing rest for the patient's caregiver. This care is paid for by the day and is all-inclusive. *Level 4* care is more intense, for patients who may require admission to a hospital or a hospice inpatient facility for a short period for management of complicated symptoms, or for end-stage management. This is the highest level of reimbursement and is paid on a per diem basis, regardless of the amount of care provided (Field & Cassel, 1997).

Although most of the financial support for hospices is provided by Medicare reimbursements, some employer-sponsored private health insurance plans, whether managed care or other forms, incorporate hospice benefits. A study by the Minnesota Hospice Association indicated that about 77% of patients enrolled in hospice were covered by Medicare, 12% by private insurance, 4% by Medicaid, and 7% from other sources (Field & Cassel, 1997). Most hospices provide some care for nonpaying, medically indigent patients, and therefore are somewhat dependent on charitable funding.

SETTINGS AND RECIPIENTS OF HOSPICE CARE

Hospice care is provided predominantly in patients' residences. However, hospice staff may visit patients in hospitals who are being referred for hospice care. In some instances, when a dying patient requires 24–hour care that cannot be provided at home, placement in a nursing care facility may be necessary. Hospice, however, may still assume overall responsibility for the patient, with support and assistance of the facility staff. Some hospices have developed a hospice house that provides facilities for hospice care for those who no longer can be cared for at home, or who may be transferred there from a hospital or nursing home.

In 1995, 77% of hospice patients died in their own personal residence, 19% in an institutional facility, and 4% in other settings (National Hospice Organization, 1998), reflecting the fact that most of those receiving hospice care were at home. In contrast, among Americans overall, 75% die in institutions—56% in hospitals and 19% in nursing homes (National Center for Health Statistics, 1998).

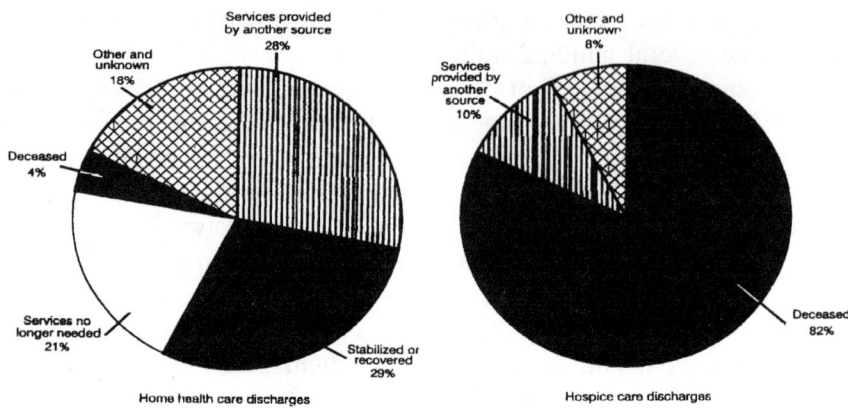

FIGURE 5.1 Discharges from home health care and hospice, 1994–1995. *Source:* Advance Data. (1998a).

Although the bulk of hospice care is provided in the home, the clientele and other characteristics of hospice agencies are substantially different from those of home health care agencies. About half of home health care patients receive care from for-profit agencies. In contrast, the vast majority of hospice care patients, over 85%, are served by not-for-profit agencies. As one might expect given the mission of hospices, death is the reason for about 82% of hospice discharges (see Figure 5.1). In sharp contrast, only 4% of home health discharges are due to the patient having died.

The MHB was based on the notion of people staying at home to die, rather than being referred to hospice just before death. On the contrary, the average length of stay in hospices nationwide has recently declined to about 12 to 18 days (National Hospice Organization, 1998). With the development of technologies prolonging life, often via home health care, hospices are receiving patients much later in their terminal illnesses. This presents problems in providing needed support for dying patients, and with hospice patient volume and associated financial challenges. This type of late intervention is, in effect, "brink of death" care or crisis management, as compared with a consistent delivery of hospice care.

As one would expect, hospice patients and other home care patients differ with respect to the frequency distribution of diagnoses. Table 5.1 shows that for home health care patients, the most common primary diagnosis is a disease of the circulatory system, most often heart disease. Other frequent diagnoses are diseases of the musculoskeletal and connective tissue, diabetes mellitus, respiratory illnesses, and injury and poisoning. Diseases of the nervous system are often listed as secondary diagnoses. In comparison, the most common primary diagnosis for hospice care patients is a malignant neoplasm or cancer (about 38%). Other frequent diagnoses are diseases of the cardiovascular system and diseases of the nervous system).

Fifty percent of all patients dying of cancer die in a hospice program, and an increasing number of aged patients with nonmalignant terminal illnesses are taking advantage of the Medicare hospice benefit (National Hospice Organization, 1998). As hospices have increased and grown, access to hospice care has been widened to include patients with congestive heart failure, chronic obstructive lung disease (COPD), AIDS, and Alzheimer's disease (Kinzbrunner, 1998). These patients have a different course of disease than do patients with cancer. They experience periods near death, only to rebound and become stable, sometimes for long periods of time (Field & Cassel, 1997). Although the stable periods are welcomed, the up-and-down clinical course makes the task of prognosis much more difficult. These patients may live longer than the 6-month period ordinarily prescribed for reimbursement. During the 1990s hospices had about 8% of patients living longer than 1 year, and about 15% of patients survived longer than 6 months (National Hospice Organization, 1998). This meant that 77% of patients died within 6 months or less. Four of five hospice care discharges occurred because of the death of the patient (Advance Data, 1998a).

In 1996, 55% of patients receiving hospice home care were female,

Table 5.1 Percent of Hospice and Home Care Patients With Certain Diagnoses or Conditions

	Hospice (%)	Home care (%)
Malignant neoplasm	37.6	2.8
Circulatory diseases	19.4	28.9
Heart disease	10.9	12.1
Respiratory disease (COPD)	6.7	2.3
Musculoskeletal-connective tissue diseases	2.9	9.0
Diabetes	2.2	7.6
Injury and poisoning	0.0	4.1

Source: Advance Data. (1998b).

compared to 45% men. The majority of patients were age 85 years or older and female. Eighty-four percent of all patients were White, and 10% were African-Americans or members of other racial or ethnic minority groups. Forty% of the patients were married. Of those who were not married, 64% were widows or widowers. Men were more likely to be married than were women, while women were more likely to be widowed. Most of the hospice care patients (78%) were living in a private or semiprivate residence, and 11% were residents of an inpatient health facility. Of the noninstitutionalized patients, 79% lived with family members, 4% lived alone, and 7% lived only with nonfamily. Women were more likely to live alone. Most patients had a primary caregiver. However, men were more likely than women both to have a caregiver and to live with their caregiver. More men than women had a spouse as their primary caregiver. Women were more likely to be cared for by a child or a child-in-law. Most of the patients received nursing services, social services, medications, and counseling. Along with volunteer services, patients received paid homemaker services. Attention by a hospice chaplain/clergy was a frequent service (Advance Data, 1998a).

According to section 418.62 of the Medicare Hospice Benefit: "A hospice must demonstrate respect for an individual's rights by ensuring that an informed consent form that specifies the type of care and services that may be provided as hospice care during the course of the illness has been obtained for every individual . . . or representative . . ." (U.S. Codes of Federal Regulations, 1993). That means that each patient and their caregiver must be informed by their physician that they are deemed terminally ill with 6 months to live, and they agree to palliative rather than curative or life-prolonging care. This is one explanation for the few pediatric patients in hospices; parents frequently do not want to "give up" the possibility that their child might recover.

HOSPICE SERVICES

Most hospice services are provided by interdisciplinary teams—nurses, social workers, home health aides, volunteers, clergy, and physicians. The family, or caregiver, of course, is involved in the individual's care as much as possible.

The hospice team has no firmly established hierarchy. This differs from almost all other health care systems, which have one profession in charge (usually physicians), even though a variety of professionals work together. The patient's principal physician must refer the patient to hospice and is always consulted throughout the course of care. But the hospice team members are dependent on each other, with the family as primary providers of care. Boundaries between members of the team are blurred, and this lack of rigidity allows for a more complete picture of the patient and the family care needs (Connor, 1998).

In most instances the patient's primary physician continues to direct patient care. Unfortunately, some physicians are reluctant to refer to hospice because they have felt financially threatened by a hospice assuming care of their patients (Field & Cassel, 1997). Direct involvement of the patient's primary physician, however, is desirable because it provides for continuity of care. The physician has principal contact with the responsible hospice nurse and social worker.

Hospices may appoint or identify a physician as a medical director, who provides certification for the admission of a patient to the hospice. The medical director may also provide education and training for nurses, social workers, students, clergy, and other volunteers; undertake utilization review, quality assurance, and ethical guidance; assume administrative responsibilities; and conduct clinical research. The medical director can review clinical information provided by the referring physician. Most hospice patients are at home under the direct care of their personal physician. However, if there is a hospice house or designated facility providing resident and/or inpatient terminal care, the medical director will be more actively involved in serving as the patient's physician.

A hospice serves as a case manager for each patient. This responsibility is largely assigned to the hospice nurse and social worker. The nurse develops and implements the majority of the care plans and coordinates visits of home health aides, social workers, and chaplains. The nurse is also responsible for ordering needed durable medical equipment, medications, and medical supplies and for maintaining close communication with the patient's primary physician and/or the hospice medical director. This might include arranging for hospitalization or respite care for symptom management, arranging transportation, and transferring information to the receiving facility (Connor, 1998).

The nurse is expected to function as the sensor for symptom management and for psychosocial needs. He or she must be well versed in opioid pain management and signs and symptoms of opioid toxicity, as well as specific therapies for anxiety, depression, nausea, constipation, and other major symptoms. In addition, the nurse is responsible for most of the patient and caregiver education regarding medications and signs and symptoms to be expected as the underlying disease progresses and the patient nears death. Hospice nurses must be available 24 hours a day, 7 days a week. The intensity of services required, including the need for continuous care of the patient in the home in the final days of life, must be determined by the nurse. In short, the hospice nurse must weave a tapestry of care from the threads of patient/family desires and the talents of the interdisciplinary team. Since 1994 a voluntary certification examination has been offered by the National Board for Certification of Hospice and Palliative Nurses in affiliation with the Hospice and Palliative Nurses Association. By the end of 1998 there were approximately 5,000 certified hospice nurses in the United States (Conner, 1998).

The hospice social worker or counselor provides psychological counseling according to the needs of the patient and family (Connor, 1998). When a family member is diagnosed with a terminal illness, the patient and the entire family are profoundly affected. The sense of loss is great and the anticipation of loss significant. Social workers help the patient and family face difficult questions about stopping treatment or life support. They can also help deal with unfinished business or financial matters and provide access to community resources, including questions about insurance, Medicare and Medicaid, Meals on Wheels, living wills, funeral planning, and other practical issues.

Spiritual support is a hallmark of hospice care, placing value on the importance of acknowledging not only physical and emotional needs, but one's spiritual or religious needs as well. This is important to many dying persons if their life is to have had meaning and purpose. The fear of death, anger at God, and fears of what may lie beyond this life are questions that dying patients may face. Hospice community or local clergy can assist patients in their life review and help them find meaning in the life they have lived. However, it is not the role of hospice to proselytize to patients about religion. The hospice chaplain can offer prayer, meditations, and support for patients requesting specific traditions, and will contact clergy to provide this support as needed. The chaplain may also assist hospice staff, and volunteers in coping with the loss of patients. Memorial services for surviving family members, staff and volunteers can be held to acknowledge and honor patients they have served.

Although public funding for hospice care has been available for some years, volunteers continue to be essential contributors to the work of hospice. Among home health care providers, the extensive use of volunteers is unique to hospice. Medicare requires that a hospice program have sufficient volunteers to provide the equivalent of at least 5% of total paid patient care hours (U.S. Codes of Federal Regulations, 1993). Over 96,000 volunteers contributed approximately 5.25 million hours of hospice service in 1992 (National Hospice Organization, 1998). Most hospices employ a volunteer coordinator who arranges for hospice volunteers to receive an average of 22 hours of instruction in hospice care. The coordinator attends meetings of the hospice team to assist volunteers in addressing patient needs. Volunteers are screened to ensure that they have no special agenda that would diverge from the care provided by hospice. Volunteers must be sensitive to end-of-life issues, including recognition of spiritual and emotional needs and appreciation of physical suffering. They may provide practical assistance in the home, or when the patient is in a hospice facility, by sitting with the patient, feeding, providing transportation, running errands, and assisting with some aspects of bedside care. Volunteers can assist in fund raising, which is especially important to not-for-profit hospices providing much charity care.

ONGOING CHALLENGES

Hospice care in the United States has developed substantially since the first hospice was established in 1971. Yet there are ongoing challenges in this field of palliative and supportive care.

Much too often, physicians are reluctant to prescribe large doses of narcotics to dying (or other) patients experiencing needless suffering. In part, this reluctance may be attributed to doctors' concerns about accusation (and conviction) of abuse and excessive use or misuse of narcotics and other registered drugs.

Palliative medicine is not yet recognized as a subspecialty in the United States, nor is it likely to be in the foreseeable future (Dockery, 1997). Few training programs in palliative medicine currently exist, and the deficiencies in training of physicians in hospice/palliative care in the United States have been critically noted (Billings & Block, 1997; Walsh, 1998). Physicians can be certified, however, by the American Academy of Hospice and Palliative Medicine.

In addition, physicians may be reluctant to refer patients who are terminally ill for hospice care. As noted at the outset of this chapter, this seems to reflect a lack of knowledge or understanding of what hospice care is, an unwillingness to discuss with patients and their families the fact that the patient is dying, and an unreasonable concern about losing their patient (Field & Cassel, 1997). Educating physicians about hospice care is a continuing need.

At the same time, patients who are dying of a terminal illness, and their families, seem generally unaware of the benefits of hospice care. Perhaps this can be attributed to the relative newness of hospice care in the United States. But it seems more likely that Americans have yet to have a rational understanding and acceptance of mortality. Elizabeth Kubler-Ross began a public discussion of these matters some three decades ago with her book *On Death and Dying* (Kubler-Ross, 1969), in which she promoted patient empowerment and home care for the terminally ill. She testified before the U.S. Senate Special Committee on Aging in 1972 and stated: "[W]we live in a very particular death-denying society. We isolate both the dying and the old, and it serves a purpose. They are reminders of our own mortality. We should not institutionalize people. We can give families more help with home care and visiting nurses, giving families and patients the spiritual and financial help in order to facilitate care at home" (Billings & Block, 1997, p. 3).

Unquestionably, social debate and discussion of death and dying will increase, especially as the very old and frail population increases, and as medical care and technology increasingly demonstrate the power to prolong life, even when characterized by suffering and total incapacity. In recent years, Dr. Jack Kevorkian has publicly advocated and practiced "physician-assisted suicide" for terminally ill patients who wish to end their irreversible suffering. And, in 1998, physician-assisted suicide became legal in the state of Oregon. These developments have led to increased discussion of palliation and hospice care as alternatives to assisted suicide.

Hospice care may also receive greater attention as the cost of medical care and its associated technology continue to present major societal and personal burdens. Current Medicare and Medicaid expenditures on the seriously and terminally ill are a growing governmental concern, and such expenditures are projected to be far greater in the decades ahead as the baby boom cohort reaches the ranks of old age. Employers who provide health insurance coverage are also concerned with the costs of persons who become seriously and terminally ill, a factor in the steady erosion of retiree health benefits offered to employees (Scanlon, 1998). As these concerns continue to grow, there may be greater attention to hospice care when it is an appropriate alternative. Little research has been done to identify how hospice care might be made less costly than it is. Moreover, sophisticated analyses of the comparative costs of hospice and more conventional medical care will be needed. In the context of such analyses, the substantial involvement of "free services" from volunteers and family members in hospice care would seem to be an important factor.

Finally, hospice may serve as an important beacon for restoring the caring component to medicine and health care more generally in the United States. It must not be overlooked that, in addition to the terminally ill, there are many who have chronic progressive diseases that prevent them from working or carrying out many activities of daily living. The course of illness in these patients may be protracted, yet be associated with increasing suffering and disability. They may not be terminally ill for years, but still are in need of the kind of supportive and compassionate care at home that is now provided by hospice to the terminally ill. Attention must be given to providing these patients with such care, which not only could improve the quality of their lives, but also decrease their dependency on costly medical care and technology.

REFERENCES

Advance Data. (1998a, August 28). *Vital and Health Statistics/CDC and Prevention/National Center for Health Statistics* (No. 299).

Advance Data. (1998b, April 16). *Vital and Health Statistics/CDC and Prevention/National Center for Health Statistics* (No. 297).

American Hospice Association. (1999). http//:www.nahc.org/haa/history.html.

Billings, J. (1998). The hospice Medicare benefit: An appraisal at 15 years— introduction to a series. *Journal of Palliative Medicine, 1*(2), 123–125.

Billings, J. A., & Block, S. (1997). Palliative care in undergraduate medical education: Status report and future directions. *Journal of the American Medical Association, 278*, 733–738.

Commission on the Future Structure of Veterans' Health Care. (1991). *Proceedings.* Washington, DC: U.S. Government Printing Office.

Connor, S. (1998). *Hospice: Practice, pitfalls, and promise.* Washington, DC: Taylor and Francis.

Dockery, J. L. (1997, February). *Palliative medicine ... What is its role in today's medical environment?* Paper presented at the meeting of the American Academy of Hospice and Palliative Medicine, Chicago, IL.

Field, M. J., & Cassel, C. K. (Eds.). (1997). *Approaching death: Improving care at the end of life.* Washington, DC: National Academy Press.

Health Care Financing Administration (1998). Medicare and Medicaid statistical supplement, 1998. *Health Care Financing Review.*

Kinzbrunner, B. (1998). Hospice: 15 years and beyond in the care of the dying. *Journal of Palliative Medicine, 1*(2), 127–137.

Kubler-Ross, E. (1969). *On death and dying.* New York: Macmillan.

Mahoney, J. (1998). The Medicare hospice benefit—15 years of success. *Journal of Palliative Medicine, 1*(2), 139–146.

National Center for Health Statistics. (1998). *New study of patterns of death in the United States* (National Mortality Followback Survey, provisional data, 1993). Bethesda, MD: Author.

National Hospice Organization. (1998, January). *Hospice Fact Sheet.*

Palmetto Government Benefit Administrators: Medicare Advisory. (1997, September). Hospice provisions enacted by the Balanced Budget Act (BBA) of 1997. *Hospice 97–11.*

Scanlon, W. J. (1998). *Retiree health insurance: Erosion in retiree health benefits offered by larger employers* (testimony before the Subcommittee on Oversight, Committee on Ways and Means, U.S. House of Representatives, March 10. GAO/T-HEHS-98-110). Washington, DC: U.S. Government Printing Office.

Stoddard, S. (1992). *The hospice movement.* New York: Vintage Books.

U.S. Code of Federal Regulations. (1993). *Medicare hospice regulations, part 418.*

Walsh, D. (1998). The Medicare hospice benefit: A critique from palliative medicine. *Journal of Palliative Medicine, 1*(2), 147–149.

CHAPTER 6

Home Care as a Business

Robert D. Hutson

Home care is the fastest growing segment in the U.S. health care industry (Leavenworth, 1995). Among the factors that have led to this growth are the expansion of Medicare benefits, lower costs for care in the home compared to hospital care, and advances in technology. Another factor has been that managed care organizations seek to discharge patients from hospital stays as swiftly as possible (Freeman, 1995). (See chapter 1 for a more detailed discussion of growth in the home care arena.)

For those persons and entities engaged in some form of the home health field of operations, home care is a business. Today, the central issue for the home care business is, Can we make it work?

There have been so many changes in the delivery of home health care in the past decade, however, that the "we" that make up the industry is constantly shifting. One can read any of the trade journals or other publications printed each month and find articles detailing home care industry mergers, alliances, "downsizings," and "rightsizings." Yesterday's competitors are working together today. Tremendous growth has occurred in some markets, and new businesses have opened. With all of these changes occurring daily, defining who the "we" is would most likely be an exercise in futility, because, once defined, the probability is that "we" will change in the next year and become something different than "we" are today.

Even as the "we" of the business constantly shifts, so does the marketing of home care to customers. For example, Kelly Services, Inc., the Kelly Girl people, started a home care business in the 1970s as a natural extension of its temporary help business. The new division, Kelly Home Care, went about setting up operations. A short time later, the name was changed to Kelly Health Care and a few years later, to Kelly Assisted Living. Why the changes? It is reported that the first name change, from *home* to *health,* occurred primarily because of a misunderstanding of the "home care" part of the name. Too much time was consumed explaining to potential customers that Kelly was not in the home repair business and did not have personnel to repair leaky gutters and broken water pipes. The next change, to Kelly Assisted Living, probably more accurately reflected the change in the company's business focus to personal type care.

In the context of such transformation, the primary purpose of this chapter is to outline strategies and approaches for ensuring the success of a home care from a business perspective in the rapidly changing home health environment. Before doing so, however, it is necessary to provide a brief overview of the business.

MAJOR HOME CARE BUSINESS SEGMENTS

The major home care business segments include Medicare-certified home health care, continuous care/personal care, home medical equipment and respiratory care, home infusion therapy, and other services.

The Medicare-certified home health care segment includes intermittently delivered skilled nursing care, physical therapy, speech therapy, occupational therapy, medical social work, and home health aide services. Patients are admitted into certified home care for intermittent care of an acute condition that usually requires treatment for a relatively short duration (typically 90 days or less). The federal Medicare program pays for these services for Medicare-eligible patients if they are homebound and require a skilled service (nursing, physical, or speech therapy), and if the service is prescribed under the direction of a physician. (Categories of persons eligible for Medicare are persons age 65 and older, those of any age who have been receiving federal disability insurance for at least

2 years, and persons who have end-stage renal disease.) This is the most common type of home care service provided. A home health agency is described as "Medicare-certified" because the Health Care Financing Administration (which administers Medicare) has deemed it as qualified to provide such services and to receive reimbursement from Medicare for providing them. These agencies also receive reimbursement from other payers such as insurance companies, the federal/state Medicaid program, employers, and others. Typically, however, 90% or greater of total revenue in these agencies is paid by Medicare.

Continuous care/personal care, often referred to as "private duty services," provides patients with an array of service capabilities. The acuity levels for care span a broad spectrum in this area. Needed services may range from a highly trained specialty nurse to a much lesser trained companion/sitter. The amount of service time spent may be as little as a few hours a month to 24 hours a day. Medicare rarely pays for this type of service.

Another segment of home care is home medical equipment (frequently referred to as durable medical equipment) and respiratory therapy services/devices. This aspect of the business supplies medical equipment such as hospital beds, ventilators, oxygen systems, wheelchairs, and prosthetic devices to patients in the home. Almost any medical device available to hospitals, nursing homes, and other institutional health care facilities can be located and provided in the home. Much of this equipment requires little training to use, but frequently it is a tool or device used by a caregiver.

Home infusion or intravenous therapy in the home is a business segment that continues to expand. Pharmaceutical products and services such as antibiotic therapies, pain management, chemotherapy, and parenteral and enteral nutrition, as well as different blood products, are provided in the home. Before 1980, almost none of these services would have even been considered for provision outside a controlled environment such as a hospital. Today, they are commonplace in the care of patients at home. The evolving technology of this industry has probably done more to enable patients to go home sooner from the hospital than any other segment of home care. This segment is often complemented by many of the other service components of home care. Customers requiring this service are frequently patients with comparatively high levels of acuity.

In addition to the above home care business segments, other services

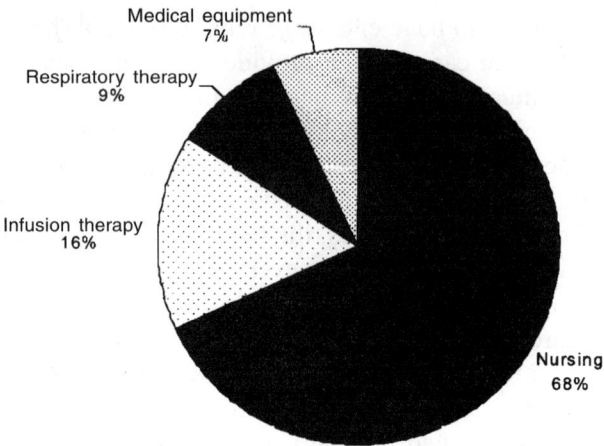

FIGURE 6.1. Home care market segments.
Source: UBS Securities (1996).

provided include fetal monitoring at home, specialty blood products, and product line "carve outs" in which patients with a particular disease or condition are targeted through services and products that are particularly relevant for them, for example, a biotech drug. Home care is playing a large role in disease-state management programs in which the caregivers are monitoring and providing care to patients in the home, whereas a few years ago this type of care would have been provided in an institution and at higher cost. There are companies today that specialize in disease-state management and contract with insurance companies to manage specific patient populations, mostly with home care services. Home care in many ways is a continuously evolving industry from a smaller cottage-type business.

Of the services provided by a home care agency, nursing services encompass the largest segment of home health care (see Figure 6.1). According to a research report (UBS Securities, 1996), nursing services account for an estimated 68% of this market segment. Infusion has grown from less than 1% in 1980 to 16% of the industry, leaping over medical equipment and respiratory therapy. Tremendous growth in the home nursing segment should continue to occur, but, for this to happen, cost inefficiencies will have to decline. In order to remain competitive and survive the prospective payment system mandated for Medicare home health services by the Balanced Budget Act of 1997, home care agencies must become more cost-effective. Achievement of cost-effectiveness will be a key component for survival of the industry as managed care squeezes reimbursement amounts.

Just a few years ago, it was commonly accepted in the industry that companies providing the full array of home care services would be the most successful, both clinically and financially. Clinically, a one-stop shop approach would provide patients with coordinated continuity of care, which enhances the quality of care. Financial success would be strengthened for a full-service agency that is able to secure an exclusive managed care contract. Home care agencies can retain profitable margins by "leveraging incremental volume over fixed investments" (UBS Securities, 1996, p. 8). Overhead costs, such as billing and collecting, decrease in larger contracts. The one-stop operational approach was widely accepted as the optimal organizational design in 1996.

Yet the industry saw many contracts with managed care firms severed in 1998, with rumors that some of the major nationwide arrangements would terminate in 1999. Although the one-stop design holds many opportunities, for many reasons achieving this optimal design with the expected positive outcomes was an overwhelming challenge in the late 1990s. From a business perspective, it was a significant effort just to keep up with all of the changes required from the various payer sources. Many organizations that were rapidly moving toward the one-stop provider status had to refocus on their core business to keep it viable; consequently, they postponed or eliminated further growth in other product lines.

TOP ADMINISTRATIVE CHALLENGES

In March 1996 the management team of Shands HomeCare, a statewide comprehensive home care operation owned by Shands HealthCare at the University of Florida, was surveyed regarding the top challenges facing home care management. The following is a composite of the perceived challenges by major category revealed in this survey (Hutson, 1996).

Managed Care

Managed care will be a norm in the health care industry. Certified home health care agencies now face shifting from a cost-reimbursed model to a discounted fee-for-service managed care mindset. Home health care agencies will find high expectations of quality and accountability but low reimbursement. Payer sources will set limitations. Managed care will enforce decreased dollars per visit.

Recruitment and Retention of Personnel

A high-quality, dedicated staff is a priority for home health care agencies. Finding top-caliber employees can be difficult. Home health care agencies face many staffing issues such as finding competent staff in rural areas, staffing employees during evenings and weekends, balancing staff and volume of business, and finding suitably experienced staff for complex cases.

Staff Development and Training

Education and critical decision-making are key in home health care. Caregivers are faced with the philosophy of "make the patient as independent as quickly as possible." Patients with higher acuity levels are being treated in the home due to earlier hospital discharges. In turn, caregivers must make critical decisions about care in an evolving reimbursement environment that includes an insurance company's case managers who tightly control the utilization of services. There also remains the constant challenge of training employees who in many cases are part-time and may work for several different organizations in the same capacity. It is common for many dollars to be spent in training and development on an employee who walks out the door several weeks or months after training. This creates a cost-effectiveness issue.

Marketing

Home health care agencies are finding it difficult to position the company with the many different consumers of the business in a positive framework (i.e., low cost, high-quality service with optimal outcomes) while working with the various payer sources. There are many conflicting demands on the home care company from its different customers. Primary customers include the patient and family, the physician, the payer, and others such as referral sources.

Financial Management

Controlling cost is a balancing act in a home health care agency, as it is in many businesses. Often the agency is asked to "do more with less." Appropriate cost accounting by service area, to calculate true cost, is challenging. So much of what is provided to the patient is a collaborative effort from an array of providers of care and service. Consequently, applying costs accurately to specific functions is difficult. (This challenge will be discussed in greater detail below.)

Information Management

Maintaining communication with staff is an ongoing process. That process becomes difficult as an agency grows and expands not only in service products but also geographically. Payers want to see outcome data regarding the cost-effectiveness of home care, so agencies are seeing the need to find ways to collect and analyze data to provide feedback to managed care organizations and to the agency itself. Proper information management and flow are seen as critical areas for the future of reducing costs in home care.

Regulatory Requirements

Federal and state governments, along with other regulatory and accrediting groups, continue to impose regulations and new requirements that drive up costs within a home health care agency. However, total reimbursement for services continues to decline. Home health care management must remain detail oriented in order to comply with regulatory issues.

Other Challenges

Other challenges facing home care management teams include coping with paperwork, getting doctors to sign necessary paperwork in a timely fashion, and addressing ethical issues when patient needs conflict with payer demands. Moreover, there has been little research conducted proving the financial value of home care.

The above synopsis of the Shands survey reveals a host of challenges a home care business faces daily. In the quest for the identification of the priority challenges to be addressed, managers have different opinions. Yet all believe that special attention to cash flow and strategic planning are essential ingredients for success in home care today.

MANAGED CARE'S ROLE IN HOME HEALTH CARE

Managed care has become a major focal point in the home health care industry. The near future of the health care system may rest in the hands of managed care, which may become the gatekeeper. Forty-one percent of the American population is covered by some type of managed care plan, whether a health maintenance organization (HMO), a preferred provider organization (PPO), or a point of service organization (PSO). Along with that growth, is the growth in enrollees of Medicare managed care (Fazzi & Agoglia, 1996).

A study conducted by the National Association for Home Care (NAHC) surveyed a cross section of managed care companies to learn their thoughts on future home care involvement (see Figure 6.2). Forty percent of those surveyed felt home care would have a 10% or higher involvement than currently. Twenty-two percent surveyed felt a 1 to 5% higher involvement would occur. Another twenty-two percent felt a 6% to 10% increased involvement would occur. However, only 4% felt that home care involvement would be the same or less than today (Fazzi & Agoglia, 1996). There is a definite shift of care from hospital to home in order to achieve efficient cost-saving patient care.

Managed care companies are looking for home health care agencies that can provide quality health services. These companies are placing emphasis on the importance of home health care agencies being accredited by a group such as the Joint Commission on Accreditation of Health Care Organizations (JCAHO). Accreditation shows that home care agencies are abiding by quality standards. Managed care organizations want agencies to provide data on their clinical outcomes and patient satisfaction. In addition to the key factors identified in the NAHC survey, home care agencies need to provide a full package of services, have critical pathways of care developed, and be proactive with patient education programs that support self-care.

Managed care organizations are also encouraging fewer and shorter visits (Fazzi & Agoglia, 1996). In accordance with this, home care indus-

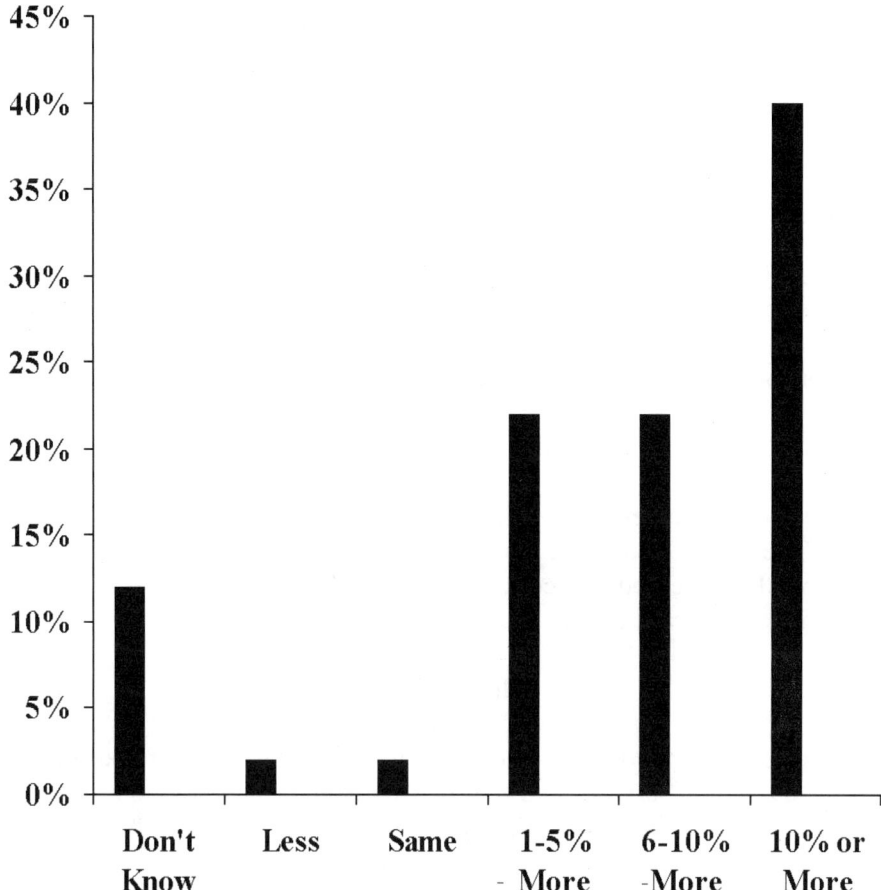

FIGURE 6.2 Managed care companies projection of involvement with home care in two years.
Source: Fazzi & Agoglia (1996).

try leaders have recognized a decrease in the number of visits per patient in all managed care arenas. Due to the decrease in visits, the overall utilization of home care agencies by managed care payers is increasing. Therefore, an increase in referrals to home care is occurring, but the overall consumption of services by individual patients is decreasing.

Home health care agencies should align themselves with managed care companies to obtain the contracts. With the emphasis being drawn away from traditional fee-for-service Medicare and placed on managed care plans, the Medicare-certified home health industry needs to address needed organizational changes.

STRATEGIES FOR SUCCESS

Stephen Tweed and Alfred Weber (1995) developed critical measures for home health care agencies to use for addressing their continued success. These measures are customer satisfaction, market share, quality-in-fact, process outcomes, and financial results.

Customer Satisfaction

To measure customer satisfaction, a numerical scale survey form can be used. The survey should be conducted both with patients and all referral sources. Two methods of collecting the information are telephone surveys or mail surveys.

Market Share

Market share in the health care arena is defined as "the number of patients an agency services and the total number of patients served in the community or agency's service area" (Tweed & Weber, 1995, p. 66). Although this can be difficult to track due to fragmentation in the home health care industry, it is possible to use national and/or regional figures and compare these numbers with agency performance.

Quality-in-fact

Measuring patient outcomes will be a vibrant concern of managed care and all accreditation organizations. Home health care agencies will use these outcomes as an integral part of defining quality-in-fact. Patient outcomes "define the desired level of function or health status at the end of a period of care" (Tweed & Weber, 1995, p. 66). To succeed in the managed care world, home health care agencies need to provide hard data indicating measurable patient outcomes at low cost. (For a detailed discussion of patient outcomes and costs, see the chapter by Shaughnessy.)

Process Outcomes

To improve a process, an agency must first measure the amount of volume derived from a process. Once measured, a quality team must work on increasing the results.

Financial Results

A vital need for agency success is the understanding of revenues, expenses, and profits. In order to keep in step with an ever-growing home health care industry, an agency must achieve adequate capital growth and have a defined financial picture. Without adequate capital growth, a home care agency will not keep up with the health care industry and its survival will be at risk.

In addition to these five areas of measurement, six strategies for success have been identified by Tweed and Weber (1995, pp. 66–67) to aid home health care agencies in managing a successful business. Those strategies are as follows:

1. Define critical measures of success. The five areas of measurement should be used to determine which specific numerical indicators will be used to measure the success of an agency.
2. Develop systems to gather the necessary information. Complete, accurate, timely information is important to this process. Health care providers must be carefully prepared for the important task of gathering, storing, analyzing, and reporting the information.
3. Display critical measures of success in graph form. Most health care professionals are "people" people, not "numbers" people. An agency's health care providers will be more likely to understand the critical measure if the numbers can be creatively displayed in the form of charts and graphs.
4. Build critical measures of success into monthly management meetings and employee communication. Displaying graphs and using them to generate discussion facilitate communication in an organization. An agency's critical measures of success can be the key to effective communication and continuous improvement in the agency.
5. Use total-quality teams and employee involvement to generate ideas for improvement. One of the hottest trends in home care today is total-quality management. A team is assigned to each of an agency's

critical measures, allowing team members to focus on the important data.
6. Use critical measures of success as the basis for an employee's recognition and rewards. Successes should be celebrated. Results should be displayed proudly. The organization's critical measures should be linked to departmental and individual performance appraisal.

The above strategies really bring together the main ingredients necessary to build success. In addition to these strategies, it is important to employ strong accounting principles.

PROPER ACCOUNTING PRINCIPLES

For a home health care agency to be successful in an era of managed care and capitation, a new form of cost accounting—*activity-based cost accounting*—should be adopted. Traditionally, cost accounting has not applied cost to activities or causes of resource consumption. (For a detailed analysis of resource consumption, see chapter 7.) With activity-based cost accounting, a four-tiered cost hierarchy is used to match resources to activities. Resources consist of cost of staff, medical supplies, health benefits, seminars, legal fees, and all other expenses associated with the operation of a home health care agency. These general ledger expenses are reclassified into activities. Then, a cost objective can be attributed to the actual cost of the activity that was performed to provide a service. Cost objectives can be based on what the agency is most focused on from a profitability standpoint such as payer or contract, product line, or program.

Although there are a number of publications on activity-based cost accounting, Tad McKeon (1995) has done an excellent job in capturing and explaining this activity. Below is a summation of his explanation along with additional comments.

Unit, batch, business, and enterprise-level expenses make up the four-tier hierarchy in activity-based cost accounting. *Unit-level* expenses are those associated with the direct cost of patient care. These include medical supplies, medical equipment, contact time, travel time, payroll, labor, and so on, that can be assigned to a specific patient. *Batch-level* expenses include costs incurred from admission to discharge. Billing, scheduling, records, direct nursing, supervision, and quality assurance functions are expenses included in this group. *Business-level* costs are those incurred prior to admission, during the time a patient is receiving service, and after discharge. Activities associated with a particular payer, product line, or program are business-level activities. Examples of business-level expenses are a specific manager overseeing a managed care contract or a director of nursing responsible for several payers in the skilled intermittent product lines. *Enterprise-level* expenses consist of senior management and other administrative expenses derived from managing several programs, product lines, or companies. These costs will be fixed and do not vary like unit costs, which are based on volume.

There are three benefits to activity-based cost accounting. One benefit is that an agency is able to determine a more accurate reflection of costs by using resource and "activity drivers." Agencies can identify the exact activity that caused expenses to be incurred, unlike traditional accounting, which ties all indirect expenses into one area.

Another benefit is the ability to cost clinical pathways. By using the four-tiered hierarchy, a price tag can be placed on each service in the clinical pathway. Per unit cost would be based on the type of visit or supply used in the clinical pathway, leading to a clearer idea of the cost of the clinical pathway. An agency can create a cost range by activity instead of using average cost by discipline.

Finally, an agency can benefit from activity-based cost accounting by not only getting a vertical view of costs incurred due to activities, but also a horizontal view of interrelationships within the organization. This horizontal view allows a manager to be proactive toward cost management. This eliminates damage control once expenses have occurred. A horizontal view consists of three parts: cost driver, activities, and performance measures. An agency can determine the reason activities are rendered, define smaller processes inside a large process, and analyze efforts being spent on the organizational mission. It is imperative for an agency to keep costs low while maintaining high quality of care to succeed. Therefore, all agency members must understand activities and processes, provide services within an appropriate price range, and create efficiency within the agency to be financially viable (McKeon, 1995).

As discussed earlier, certified agencies need to move away from a prevalent "Medicare-certified mindset." Under the cost-reporting requirements of Medicare, an agency does not obtain the true or correct view of costs associated with the activity. These distorted aggregate data do not reflect true cost or a strategic management plan. Lacking that accurate information, it is virtually impossible to know what cost rates should be when making contracts with payers. Regardless, if the payer is seeking a discounted fee-for-service agreement, or one where the home care agency is fully at risk financially for a given patient population through a capitation methodology, the agency will be working in the dark until it applies activity-based cost accounting.

CRITICAL PATHWAY DEVELOPMENT

Home health care is evolving into a truly active part of the health care delivery plan. No longer should home care be thought of as a carve out business or an afterthought in the continued care of a patient. However, in providing care in the home, home health care agencies are faced with providing high-quality care at a cost-effective rate. There is a need to decrease labor and material waste. As health care moves into the managed care model, it is important for home health care agencies to be able to provide outcome data and a clear, accurate prediction of care. In addition, because emphasis is placed on continuity of care between all health care providers (i.e., physicians, hospitals, home care agencies, and long-term care facilities), there is a need for an effective method of communication between these providers. A system of tracking patient outcomes, evaluating care, and providing communication among providers is through critical pathway development.

Critical pathways map out a treatment plan and provide patient goals to be achieved. By using a critical pathway, data can be collected on the process of treating a certain diagnosis, then analysis can be done on variances that have occurred. These variances are present when expected outcomes have not been realized in the scheduled time frame of the critical pathway. Patient goals achieved ahead of schedule are considered to be positive variances. Those variances that result due to the fact that achievement of patient goals is behind the scheduled time frame are considered negative variances. Once analysis has been completed on the variances, fine-tuning of the critical pathway can take place by revising or further developing the pathway. Home health care agencies are able to use this information to continually improve quality of patient care.

Benefits can be seen by using critical pathways. In a study of one home health care agency (Maturen & Van Dyck, 1996), some of the benefits recognized by staff and managers were improved time management, improved documentation, improved consistency with policies and procedures, and improved assessment of staff education needs, patient teaching needs, and support materials. Administrators also noted improvements in projection and tracking of resource utilization, facilitation of program development, and support of marketing efforts. By welcoming the ideas behind critical pathways and becoming proactive in the ever-changing health care environment, home care agencies can successfully meet challenges, changes, and trends.

Critical pathways also have distinct advantages in the mapping of patient care. Many of the ingredients to the pathway are concrete activities that are local custom. Negative variances are significant issues that need to be addressed. It is readily acceptable that a certain percentage of patients will "fall off" their designed critical pathway. What is not addressed very well is how the care team should pick up a patient's care when he or she falls off the pathway. Combining activity analysis with critical pathways adds valuable information for the care team.

SOME FURTHER OBSERVATIONS

The aim of this chapter was to look at some of the major issues and challenges facing the business segment of home care today. It also was to give some structure and organization to thoughts about how "we" can make it work.

One topic touched on but not discussed in any detail is the role of information management. It almost can go without saying that to be successful in the home care business, a strong information management system is required. Selecting the right system to meet an agency's needs is probably as important as the use of a system itself. Telemedicine and other technological advances will continue to enable new capabilities in this area (see chapter 3).

Reimbursement strategies are very difficult to track, but they are essential to agency survival. With the continual changes in how the Health Care Financing Administration (HCFA) governs Medicare dollars, an entire book could be written on the subject but be outdated before going to press. HCFA's present implementation of an interim payment system for home care on the way to its adopting a prospective payment system has created more turmoil in the certified agencies business than anything in the industry's history. Many in the home care field attribute the closing of over 1,000 Medicare-certified agencies in 1998 to that initiative alone. HCFA's dramatic reduction in reimbursement for oxygen and other equipment has severely affected providers of that service. Insurance companies are focusing closely on the costs of medication and nutritional support products provided by home infusion companies and in many ways are treating them as commodity providers without much emphasis on the service component. To survive this rather dramatic assault on reimbursement for home care services, the successful providers will need to become more operationally efficient and have an accurate knowledge of their costs.

Positioning a home care company for the future has considerable challenges. Home care continues to be an integral part of the total health care delivery system. It is now recognized as one of the most essential ingredients to optimal outcomes. Agencies that do not make themselves part of a large delivery system may not survive. In the years ahead, home care will cease to be considered as an afterthought in the health care arena; those who still consider it to be an afterthought will not stay in business. The larger the providers become in their geographical area, the more economies of scale they may achieve and the better able they will be to leverage those economies to reduce costs. Demonstrated quality outcomes as measured for all customers are essential.

The term *home care* will probably stay around for a few years. However, this industry is now positioning itself as the engine for a "mobile health care delivery network," which is the next step in the health care evolution. We will see an increase in the number of patient care teams that move beyond the traditional brick and mortar of an institution to a multitude of treatment sites. Additionally, the personnel who make up these teams will work in a variety of environments rather than in a single one, as has been the custom. Institutional settings that have home care organizations may come to draw on home care operations—their medical and personnel records, as well as their administrative processes. These systems are easily transferable and can give the once rigid institutionally designed organization the flexibility to move caregivers and patients throughout the continuum of care with greater efficiency and better patient outcomes.

REFERENCES

Fazzi, R. A., & Agoglia, R. V. (1996). Managed care's expectations: Final results from a national study. *Caring, 15*(1), 10–16.

Freeman, L. (1995). Home-sweet-home health care (home health services growth). *Monthly Labor Review, 118,* 3–11.

Hutson, R. D. (1996). *Shands HomeCare management survey of top challenges facing administration in home care.* Gainesville, FL: Shands HomeCare.

Leavenworth, G. (1995). The fastest growing segment of the health care industry combines cost-effective, high-quality care with the comforts of home (home health care) [Special issue]. *Business and Health Annual,* 51–55.

Maturen, V., & Van Dyck, L. (1996). Using outcome-based critical pathways to improve documentation. *Home Health Care Management and Practice, 8*(2), 48–58.

McKeon, T. (1995). Activity-based cost management: A tool for survival. *Journal of Home Health Care Practice, 7*(4), 69–75.

National Association for Home Care. (1995). *Basic statistics about home care, 1995.* Washington, DC: Author.

Tweed, S. C., & Weber, A. J. (1995). Critical measures of success: A tool for organizational effectiveness, communication, and continuous improvement in home health care. *Journal of Home Health Care Practice, 7*(4), 64–68.

UBS Securities. (1996). *Home care industry report: Home of healthy growth.* New York: Author.

SECTION THREE

FINANCING, AUSPICES, AND QUALITY OF CARE

CHAPTER 7

Issues in Understanding Resource Consumption in Publicly Funded Home Care

Richard H. Fortinsky
Elizabeth A. Madigan

The well-documented growth of the home care industry in the United States (Branch, Goldberg, Chen, & Williams, 1993; Kane et al., 1994; Welch, Wennberg, & Welch, 1996) has led to concerns about containing home care costs—the consumption of resources—while maintaining adequate quality of care. The federal Medicare program, which finances almost half of all home care spending, recently experienced a rapid increase in total payments for such services, from $3.2 billion in 1989 to $16.8 billion in 1996 (Health Care Financing Admin-

---

The authors gratefully acknowledge the support of the Center for Community Based Care, Ohio Council for Home Care. Portions of this book chapter were presented at the 1996 Annual Meeting of the American Public Health Association. Partial support for Dr. Madigan was provided by the National Institute for Nursing Research, National Research Service Award, NR 06987-02.

istration, 1998). The number of Medicare-certified home care agencies also increased dramatically between 1980 and 1996, growing from 2,924 to 9,850 agencies in that period (Health Care Financing Administration, 1998). Similar growth in home care spending has occurred in the state/federal Medicaid program. Between 1987 and 1997, total Medicaid home care spending increased from $2.1 billion to $13.5 billion, growing from 11% to 24% of all Medicaid long-term care spending (Coleman, 1999).

Insurers, regulators, and providers of home care expect continued growth in the home care industry due to several factors. These factors include projected increases in the older and younger disabled populations over the next several decades, technological advancements allowing more skilled services to be provided in the home setting, and preferences of most patients to receive care at home rather than in institutional settings (see chapters 1, 2, and 3).

In response to cost and quality concerns associated with the rapid growth of home care, health services researchers have been helping payers and providers examine alternative approaches to financing and monitoring the quality of home care services. For example, Branch and Goldberg (1993) published results aimed at informing decision makers about how to design a prospective payment system (PPS) for Medicare home health care based on patient case mix. Such PPS systems are under active consideration by the U.S. Health Care Financing Administration (HCFA), the federal agency responsible for administering the Medicare and Medicaid programs (Clauser, 1994; Hoyer, 1995; Ingoldsby, Kumar, Cohen, & Wallack, 1994; Schlenker, 1996). Additional studies on resource consumption by home care patients over episodes of care have informed debates about home care reimbursement options for Medicare and Medicaid (Branch et al., 1993; Goldberg & Schmitz, 1994; Swan, Black, Benjamin, & Fox, 1995).

In this chapter, we devote primary attention to the question What do we know about resource consumption in publicly funded home care, particularly in Medicare home care? Our major purpose is to highlight recent and current efforts by home care researchers and policy stakeholders to measure and explain observed trends in Medicare home care resource consumption. We also summarize ongoing efforts to develop a payment system to control home care resource consumption by Medicare beneficiaries. Current attempts to understand relationships between home care resource consumption and patient outcomes among Medicare beneficiaries also are described (see also chapter 8).

We have chosen to deal primarily with Medicare home care resource consumption in this chapter because it accounts for the greatest proportion of all home care spending and because it continues to command the attention of federal policymakers alarmed at the rapid growth of this Medicare benefit. Historically, the Medicare home care benefit has been used most widely for skilled nursing, home health aide, and rehabilitation therapy services delivered to patients to help them recuperate from acute illnesses or injuries. In contrast, home care services delivered to help persons with more chronic physical and mental health problems to delay or avoid nursing facility admission are financed by a combination of Medicaid funds, state funds, Older Americans Act funds, and in some states, county or local funds (Hegner, 1996). Despite the focus on Medicare, we note in this chapter that the distinction between Medicare home care and home care funded by other public funding sources is blurring as more patients with coexisting acute and chronic health problems enter the home care system.

We also have chosen to focus on home care resource consumption by older Americans (age 65 years or older) because they are the predominant users of home care. According to the 1996 National Home and Hospice Care Survey, older persons accounted for 72.2% of all home care patients receiving services at the time of the survey and for 66.1% of all home care patients discharged prior to the survey (these figures exclude hospice patients; Haupt, 1998). Moreover, older persons make up a larger proportion of Medicaid home care caseloads than younger disabled persons in most states (Coleman, 1999).

As a final introductory note, it is important to acknowledge that in addition to these major publicly funded sources of home care, individuals may finance home care through either out-of-pocket payments or private insurance (Levit et al., 1997). Given our focus on publicly funded home care, and Medicare home care in particular, an examination of trends in privately financed home care resource consumption is beyond the scope of this chapter.

Specific issues addressed in this chapter include:

- What eligibility criteria drive demand for publicly funded home care resource consumption?
- What is the state of the art in measuring resource consumption in home care?
- What are the known predictors of publicly funded home care re-

source consumption based on health services research and gerontological literature?
- How is home care resource consumption related to patient outcomes?
- What conclusions can be drawn, and what unanswered questions remain, concerning home care resource consumption?

ELIGIBILITY CRITERIA FOR PUBLICLY FUNDED HOME CARE

To be eligible for postacute home care under the Medicare program, a beneficiary must (1) be confined to a place of residence (known as the "homebound" provision), (2) have a plan of care approved by a physician, and (3) need part-time or intermittent skilled services, such as skilled nursing or physical therapy. So long as these criteria are met, a beneficiary also may receive home health aide services, medical social services, occupational therapy, medical supplies, and durable medical equipment (Goldberg & Schmitz, 1994).

The definitions of *homebound* and *part-time or intermittent* have been subject to much debate and legal action that has broadened their meaning in the Medicare program. In the 1989 revisions to the Medicare Health Insurance Manual (HIM-11), *homebound* was defined as requiring considerable and taxing effort for the patient to leave the home. Examples were offered to clarify who would and would not qualify under this definition (Kenney &Moon, 1997; Mauser, 1997). The HIM-11 also clarified the definition of *part-time or intermittent*" care. *Intermittent* was explicitly defined as up to 28 hours per week of skilled nursing and home health aide services, and *part-time* as 8 hours per day for up to 21 consecutive days, although both could be extended under special circumstances (Kenney & Moon, 1997). These clarifications have helped reduce inconsistencies in eligibility determinations by Medicare's 10 regional fiscal intermediaries (FIs), private organizations with which HCFA contracts to review and audit home care claims. Anecdotal evidence in the home care industry suggests that these regional FIs vary in their interpretations of nationally standardized Medicare home care eligibility criteria, yet no scientifically sound evidence has been published to support these assertions.

Eligibility requirements for Medicaid and other publicly funded home care vary from state to state, because state governments have the authority to establish eligibility criteria for in-home and community-based services intended to keep recipients at home as long as possible. The cornerstones of eligibility criteria for these services in most states are the inability of the applicant to conduct basic activities of daily living (ADLs) and instrumental activities of daily living (IADLs). Cognitive impairment and behavioral problems are also used as eligibility criteria in a majority of states. Yet there is no consensus among states regarding how these factors should be defined, measured, or combined to form quantifiable eligibility criteria. Furthermore, although all states consider applicants eligible for publicly funded home care only if they would otherwise be eligible for nursing facility placement, there is great variation among states in minimum eligibility for nursing facility placement (O'Keeffe, 1996).

Distinctions in eligibility for Medicare versus Medicaid and other publicly funded home care evolved from two different programmatic views about the intention of home care. Medicare home care was intended to help acutely ill persons recover at home, whereas Medicaid and other public programs were intended to provide long-term home care. Nevertheless, there are patients who require both sets of services, either simultaneously or sequentially. One type of patient has health conditions that exhibit patterns of remission and exacerbation over time. A second type of patient has health conditions that begin as acute problems but do not progress adequately to allow full recovery, resulting in the need for long-term home care. Finally, there are patients for whom services are initiated for an acute condition that progresses to recovery, but who require long-term home care for other diseases unrelated to the initial acute condition.

Several examples may help clarify these patient types. In the first type, patients with chronic obstructive pulmonary disease may require ongoing paraprofessional (aide or homemaker) assistance with ADLs and IADLs related to diminished lung capacity. During times when an exacerbation of the illness necessitates close observation of the condition and patient teaching related to self-care, professional nursing services would also be needed in addition to the ongoing ADL and IADL support. In the second type, some patients do not progress as expected following a fractured hip and never regain functional independence. These patients start out with physical therapy services, but once a plateau in progress has been reached, paraprofessional services are needed to provide the support for the patient to remain at home. In the third type, patients with arthritic and osteoporotic changes who are hospitalized for treatment of hypertension may require nursing care related to assessment and patient teaching for the hypertension, a long with ongoing paraprofessional ADL and IADL support related to the arthritic changes that affect the ability to function independently.

In summary, current practices in postacute and long-term home care leave room for doubt about the extent to which there are uniform eligibility criteria allowing access to either Medicare home care or Medicaid and other publicly funded home care throughout the United States. Furthermore, very little is known about the extent of demand for both types of home care by the same patients, either simultaneously or sequentially. Our knowledge about how to predict or control home care resource consumption patterns will inevitably be limited until improvements are made in determining uniform eligibility criteria for either or both types of home care.

MEASURES OF HOME CARE CONSUMPTION

In this section, we summarize various units of analysis used to measure home care resource consumption. In doing so, we focus primarily on Medicare home care, although some measures may be relevant to Medicaid home care as well. Trends indicate a movement away from the visit per se as the primary unit of interest among researchers and policymakers, and increased interest in episodes of care and visit length (time-based measures). Researchers are also becoming more creative in their uses of Medicare claims data and agency-specific data (e.g., HCFA 485 forms) to construct episodes and distinguish patterns of service delivered by different disciplines.

The Home Care Visit

A visit refers to in-home contact between a patient and a health professional or paraprofessional, without regard to time spent or type of care provided. Until very recently, the visit has been the most common unit of analysis used in home care research to describe patterns of resource consumption and to explore factors affecting variation in home care service use. Most dependent variables employed in such research are based on home visits. Common measures include whether or not a home visit was made during a study period, total number of home visits made over a study period, and number of visits adjusted for the number of users. Much of this research has examined predictors of visit-based measures against the conceptual framework of predisposing, enabling, and need characteristics of home care patients, agency characteristics, and/or characteristics of the health care system, or environment, in specific geographic areas (Andersen, 1995; Andersen & Newman, 1973). Several of these studies are summarized later in this chapter.

Historically, the visit also has been the unit of resource consumption used for payment of Medicare home care. The Medicare program has traditionally paid certified home health agencies on a retrospective cost basis, where the cost per visit is the foundation of the reimbursement formula (Mauser, 1997). Clarifications of eligibility criteria for Medicare home care implemented in 1989 via the HIM-11 not only broadened the definitions of *part-time* and *intermittent,* but also broadened the types of skilled service visits that would be covered. For example, nursing visits for the management and evaluation of a patient's care plan were covered for the first time (Kenney & Moon, 1997). Recent rapid increases in Medicare expenditures for home care resource consumption are due primarily to growth in the number of visits in response to these eligibility modifications, not to Medicare per-visit payment increases (Bishop, Brown, Phillips, Ritter, & Skwara, 1996; Cohen & Tumlinson, 1997; Hegner, 1996).

HCFA's cost-based reimbursement approach for home care visits has come under intense scrutiny, because of both escalating Medicare expenditures and administrative burdens associated with determining allowable costs (Goldberg & Schmitz, 1994). The initial phase of an ongoing PPS experiment launched in 1991 by HCFA focused explicitly on substituting cost-based reimbursement for prospectively set rates for the six major types of home health visits covered by Medicare. Results of this experiment showed that a per-visit PPS payment methodology would have little effect on costs per visit and that participating agencies did not increase their number of visits to patients, decrease quality of care, or increase patient selectivity to improve profitability (Bishop et al., 1996; Phillips, Brown, & Bishop, 1994).

The Balanced Budget Act of 1997 (BBA97) established an interim payment system (IPS) for Medicare home care. While the policy goal of the IPS is to reduce Medicare home care payments by more than $16 billion over 5 years, this new payment system remains cost-based and rests on the foundation of the home visit (Gage, Stevenson, Liu, & Aragon, 1998; National Association for Home Care, 1997). The IPS modified Medicare's home care payment method to home care agencies primarily by reducing their per-visit cost limits and by introducing an aggregate-per-beneficiary utilization limit. The latter feature does not restrict the number of visits to individual patients, but it does require agencies to balance the number of visits made to all types of Medicare home care patients throughout the fiscal year (National Association for Home Care, 1997). This current payment system reinforces the visit as the paramount measure of resource consumption in Medicare home care. It has also had the effect of making it difficult for some home care agencies to survive financially (see Gage et al., 1998, and chapter 11).

Length of the Home Care Visit

In contrast to the considerable amount of research on visits as measurement units of home care resource consumption, little evidence is available about the length of time spent by home care professionals in the home during visits. This is not surprising, because visit-based reimbursement systems have monopolized home care policy under Medicare and Medicaid. Until recently, studies examining length of visits in home care research have been restricted primarily to research on nursing productivity (Bishop et al., 1996). Nevertheless, since HCFA has begun experimenting with PPS for home care visits, interest has grown in visit length as a potential indicator of decisions made by home care agency administrators to maximize the efficiency of their operations.

Research conducted as part of the first phase of HCFA's ongoing PPS demonstration uncovered preliminary estimates of the effect of per-visit prospective payment on visit length. Visit length data were based on patient or proxy recall ($N = 2,108$ respondents) for the most recent home care visit made during the study episode. For all 47 participating home care agencies, this study found considerable variation in average visit lengths for both skilled nurses (mean = 42 minutes; range = less than 15 minutes to 8 hours) and home health aides (mean = 79 minutes; range = 15 minutes to 8 hours). Home care agencies that were paid prospectively for visits ($N = 26$) had statistically significant shorter average home health aide visits than matched control agencies ($N = 21$), even after controlling for numerous covariates. This difference was not observed, however, for skilled nursing visits. These findings strongly suggest that home health visits are not well-defined units, given the substantial variation in observed lengths of visits by both nurses and home health aides. Moreover, if per-visit prospective payment systems are put in place, home care agencies may make decisions to reduce the length of visits to reduce costs, particularly for home health aides (Bishop et al., 1996).

Length of visits in home care also is affected by the major health problem of patients and by the overall case mix of home care agencies. Payne and colleagues used a prospective design to collect data on the length of skilled nursing visits ($N = 4,426$ visits) made to a diverse sample of patients served by 12 not-for-profit home care agencies in Massachusetts (Payne, Thomas, Fitzpatrick, Abdel-Rahman, & Kayne, 1998). This study found statistically significant differences in mean length of skilled nursing visits, depending on the major health problem recorded for study patients. For example, patients with medical/surgical problems had the shortest visits (mean = 33.3 minutes), and hospice/terminally ill patients had the longest (mean = 59.5 minutes). In multivariate analyses controlling for numerous patient and visit characteristics, agency differences in mean visit length were highly statistically significant. The persistence of agency differences suggests that information beyond the case mix of agency patients is needed to understand agency decision-making processes and other factors involved in determining visit lengths.

Length of home care visits is likely to emerge as an important measure of home care resource consumption in the near future. Research is now under way to develop a model to predict home care resource consumption that includes the innovation of incorporating several variables that may affect the length of home care visits. These variables include staff changes during the episode of care and psychosocial interventions during visits (Goldberg, 1997).

Episode of Home Care

Viewing home care resource consumption from an "episode perspective" recognizes that patients receive a number of home care visits over a period of time from a potential variety of disciplines. Until recently, given the domination of the per-visit perspective in the measurement of home care resource consumption, very little health services research has focused on the episode as the unit of analysis within which to examine visit patterns or "length of stay." Now that phase 2 of HCFA's PPS demonstration project is well under way, however, interest in the home care episode as a unit of home care resource consumption has dramatically increased among providers and payers (Goldberg & Schmitz, 1994).

Episodes of care have been measured using three different sources of data: Medicare claims data (Goldberg & Schmitz, 1994; Schore, 1996), agency-specific data based on standardized forms submitted to HCFA (Branch and Goldberg, 1993; Branch et al., 1993), and patient-specific data collected prospectively, using standardized forms (Fortinsky & Madigan, 1997).

Goldberg and Schmitz (1994) explained the difficulty of defining and constructing an episode of Medicare-reimbursed home care due to the intermittent nature of service delivery, especially when claims data are used as a data source. Their definition of an episode (consistent with the HCFA per-episode PPS demonstration project) was all services delivered during a period of 120 days following initial admission. They allowed a 45–day gap between such periods before identifying new episodes of care. In contrast, Schore (1986) used Medicare claims data to construct episodes of care as periods of time "covered by strings of consecutive Medicare claims that were preceded and followed by a 30–day minimum hiatus in claims" (p. 2). A further complication is that home care agencies vary in their definition of a discharge. For example, some agencies always administratively discharge patients who become hospitalized, then consider these patients as new admissions if they begin home care again after hospital discharge. Other agencies would not consider such a patient as a discharge unless the hospitalization exceeded a minimum amount of time. Construction of episodes from claims data will always be limited by lack of information about varying definitions of discharge used by agencies whose patients are included in these databases.

In general, descriptive results of studies on episodes of home care have yielded different average lengths of episodes, depending on the source of data. Studies based on claims data have shown longer episode lengths than studies based on agency-specific data (Branch et al, 1993; Goldberg & Schmitz, 1994; Welch et al., 1996). Very little is presently known about decision-making processes within home care agencies that may influence episode lengths, or the number of visits provided during episodes. At the time of this writing, preliminary results of site visits made to home care agencies by evaluators of the HCFA phase 2 (per-episode) PPS demonstration have been submitted to HCFA for staff review (B. R. Phillips, personal communication, February 21, 1997). When released, these findings should shed light on how agencies respond to prospective payment for episodes of care.

Staff Mix

A final approach to measuring home care resource consumption involves examining the distribution of specific types of home care professionals deployed by home care providers. Patterns in staff mix can be studied in the aggregate, to determine whether specific types of staff are being used more or less commonly over time in the entire home care industry, or in cross-agency comparisons, where proportions of visits made by different disciplines can be contrasted.

National data reveal that home health aide visits increased from 33.8% of all Medicare-reimbursed home care visits in 1988, to 48.9% of all visits in 1996. Conversely, the skilled nursing visits decreased from 51.1% to 41.1% of all visits over the same period. Even more dramatic was the rise in home health aide visits per Medicare home care beneficiary, from an average of 20.9 in 1988 to an average of 73.0 in 1996. Similar figures for nursing visits per Medicare beneficiary were 13.3 and 24.4, respectively (Health Care Financing Administration, 1998). These figures indicate that home health aides have surpassed nurses as the most common Medicare home care providers. The use of both types of providers has increased on a per-beneficiary basis, but the increase in home health aide use has greatly exceeded the increase in the use of nurses.

These trends have led to growing concern that home care resource consumption patterns funded by Medicare increasingly resemble long-term home care rather than postacute care (Schore, 1996; Welch et al., 1996). However, the reliance on home health aides in Medicaid-funded and state-funded long-term home care programs is, comparatively, still much higher. For example, a study of long-term home care programs in the state of Maine revealed that 80% to 90% of total resource consumption was related to home health aide care (Fortinsky, Hathaway, & McGuire, 1992).

Very little is known about cross-agency comparisons in staff mix for home care episodes. As with length of home care visits, the staff mix dimension of home care resource consumption is expected to grow in importance as home care agencies make decisions about staff deployment in response to new payment systems such as Medicare IPS and PPS.

One recently completed study compared results when different measures of home care resource consumption are constructed over complete episodes of care using the same study sample. Number of visits, length of visits, and estimated costs per day were calculated for nurses, home health aides, therapists, and medical social workers in a sample of patients who completed an episode of home care. Although mean length of time per visit did not differ across staff types, mean number of visits and costs per day of the episode did vary considerably (Madigan & Fortinsky, 1999). This type of empirical research should stimulate replication and discussion about the relative importance of monitoring different measures of home care resource consumption as home care agencies are exposed to new payment systems.

PREDICTORS OF HOME CARE RESOURCE CONSUMPTION

Predictions of home care resource consumption can be undertaken on three levels—the patient level, the agency level, and the system (environment) level (see Andersen, 1995). The literature on this topic contains disparate definitions of home care, with some studies examining samples of Medicare home care users, and others focusing on long-term home care users. In this section, we do not distinguish between these types of home care, but instead focus on patterns of findings based on a uniform explanatory framework.

There is considerable empirical evidence that patient-level factors are most likely to explain home care resource consumption, although methodological differences among the studies complicate thorough comparisons. There is also evidence for the factors predictive of resource consumption on the agency and system levels, although this body of research is not as extensive as for the patient level. Finally, there is some preliminary work being undertaken on the interplay between the levels, although no research is currently available that examines resource consumption as a function of predictors from all three levels.

Patient-Level Predictors

Resource consumption on this level has most often been conceptualized in three ways—use or nonuse of services, the number of disciplines providing care, and the total number of visits by all disciplines. Much of the work in this area was done in the late 1970s through the mid-1980s and includes single-site as well as multisite studies. Use or nonuse of services was studied by Branch and colleagues (1981, 1988), Soldo (1985), and Solomon and colleagues (1993). The number of different disciplines or services were studied by Branch and colleagues (1988) and Evashwick, Rowe, Diehr, and Branch (1984), using the same study sample but different operational definitions of the dependent variable. McAuley and Arling (1984) used both the use or nonuse of services and the number of services, whereas Kemper (1992) and Coughlin, McBride, Perozek, and Liu (1992), studied the number of hours of formal care. Starrett, Rogers, and Walters (1989) used the total number of home care visits provided during the study period. Finally, Pasquale (1987) studied the total number of nursing visits as well as all types of visits, whereas Edwardson and Nardone (1991) studied the total number of nursing and home health aide visits.

In many of these studies the Andersen behavioral model (Andersen & Newman, 1973)—with its conceptual framework of predisposing, enabling, and need-level variables—was used to frame the selection and organization of variables for predicting measures of resource consumption. Accordingly, the 10 studies can be summarized in terms of the Anderson framework. It should be noted that the summary of variables, below, includes those most often used in the studies, but does not include a complete listing of all variables from each study.

The *predisposing* factors summarized in these studies were age, gender, and nonwhite ethnicity. In 9 of the 10 studies, age was a statistically significant predictor of home care resource consumption. Females were more likely than males to use home care services in four studies, suggesting that males relied more on spouses than on formal services for in-home assistance. Ethnicity was not a predictor of home care resource consumption in these studies.

The most important *enabling* factors across the studies were income levels and Medicaid enrollment. Home care resource consumption was found to be greater among individuals with less income, who, of course, are more likely to qualify for Medicaid and other public sources of funding for home care.

Need factors of various kinds were clear predictors of home care resource consumption. This was especially the case with respect to the Katz scale of dependence in ADLs. Other need factors included IADL scores, other functional status measures, cognitive impairment, depression, self-perceptions of health, incontinence, and dependence on medical equipment.

Overall, these studies showed that factors involving the *need* for care were more influential in predicting home care resource consumption than either *predisposing* or *enabling* factors. Regardless of the measure of resource consumption or study methodology, *functional status at admission to home care has had the most consistent predictive power.*

Agency-Level Predictors

Influences on resource consumption stemming from the home care agency level are type of agency ownership, affiliation of the agency with a larger organizational entity (vertical integration) or with other agencies or providers (horizontal integration), market factors, and home care staffing differences. This area of research is less well developed compared to studies of individual patient predictors, but certain trends are emerging.

There is evidence about differences by agency ownership (proprietary vs. not-for-profit) in patterns of home care service delivery. Not-for-profit agencies have been found to provide care to more Medicaid and indigent patients than proprietary agencies (Shuster & Cloonan, 1991). Patients served by proprietary agencies received more total visits, more visits per week, and thus higher charges than patients served by not-for-profit or governmental agencies (Williams, 1994). In work on geographic area variations in Medicare home care, Kenney and Dubay (1992) found that in areas with a higher proportion of proprietary agencies, more visits were provided. More recently, 1996 Medicare data indicate that proprietary agencies provided an average of 104 visits per patient served, whereas not-for-profit and governmental agencies provided substantially fewer services, 55 and 61 visits per patient, respectively (Health Care Financing Administration, 1998). Williams (1994) suggested that differences in service delivery are explained by the efforts of proprietary agencies pushed to maximize revenues in a cost-based reimbursement system that had few incentives to control the number of visits.

The organizational affiliations of agencies have not been studied in the same depth as ownership, although there is evidence that agencies that are vertically integrated with hospitals provide fewer visits per home care episode than nonaffiliated agencies (Goldberg & Schmitz, 1994). This difference in resource consumption is not apparently attributable to differences in the clients served, because there is evidence that home care patient case mix does not differ between hospital-affiliated and non-affiliated agencies (Pettigrew, Kramer, & Shaughnessy, 1988). Agencies that are horizontally integrated, that is, part of a chain of home care agencies, have not been studied in comparison to freestanding agencies, so it is not yet possible to draw conclusions about effects of horizontal integration on resource consumption.

Discussions of types of ownership and affiliation have not considered the interplay between the two factors, but there is preliminary evidence from national data that proprietary agencies are more likely to be horizontally integrated (Madigan, 1996). The current rapid pace of both horizontal integration and vertical integration (i.e., where home care agencies are part of multiservice health systems) is leading to greater geographical distances between home care resource consumption decision-making and the actual delivery of home care by individual agencies. Other research, however, suggests that the distinctions between types of ownership and affiliation are misleading, implying instead that the specific market concentration of agency types in a geographic area influences individual agency behavior. Estes and Swan (1994) term this institutional isomorphism, from the work by DiMaggio and Powell (1983), where agencies within a specific geographic market behave similarly with regard to resource consumption decisions regardless of ownership and affiliation types.

Several home care agency staff characteristics also bear consideration when examining resource consumption in the context of agency "predictors" of home care resource consumption. One agency characteristic that is often overlooked in empirical studies is the method of staff payment. Two common forms of payment are per-visit and per-hour pay. Per-visit payment to staff is attractive to agencies under the current fee-for-service system, because staff are paid only for visits for which payment is made to the agency. There is anecdotal evidence from the home care industry that resource consumption is higher under a per-visit payment scheme. Indeed a logical case can be made that per-visit pay engenders inefficient use of resources because it tends to maximize the number of visits per patient and ensure specific salary levels for staff. However, proposed changes in the reimbursement system for home care may make the per-visit payment scheme difficult to design and manage under a prospective, episode-based reimbursement system.

A second overlooked issue related to staff characteristics pertains to potential variations in clinical and administrative practices among staff within and between agencies. For example, new staff members may be less comfortable with or uncertain about the expected trajectory of patient progress, and may therefore order or approve more home visits to ensure that patients are being sufficiently monitored. Another possible source of variation in home care resource consumption is different philosophical stances among staff members. Some staff members may be committed to promoting maximum levels of individual or family self-care, whereas others may see their roles as more directly involved in "doing for" the patient. These staff differences in care philosophy would point to the lack of a guiding practice framework within home care agencies for determining the number of home care visits and, therefore, resource consumption.

System-Level Predictors

Numerous studies have found geographic variations throughout the United States in home care resource consumption, but it is not clear why these differences persist (Kenney & Dubay, 1992; Schore, 1996; Welch et al., 1996). In response to concerns about differences in interpretation among HCFA's 10 regional FIs regarding allowable Medicare home care services, the agency funded a study (Schore, 1996) to examine whether FI differences in interpretation explained geographic variations. This research did find geographic differences, with patients in the east-south-central part of the country receiving more than three times the visits of patients in the Pacific region, the lowest-use region. Yet differences could not be explained solely by the practices of FIs. The study indicated that patients in the higher resource consumption areas were more likely than those in other areas to have long-term care needs, and more likely to be served by proprietary agencies. The author concluded that there are numerous unmeasured factors influencing these regional differences, including local physician and home care provider practice patterns, that appear to be operating at a level greater than the individual provider.

Local and state health care market factors have been studied as system-level influences on home care resource consumption, with mixed results. Studies have found that the supply of nursing home beds in a geographic area has an inverse relationship to the proportion of patients who receive home care (Kenney & Dubay, 1992; Swan & Benjamin, 1993). In other studies comparing geographic areas, no significant association was found between hospital bed supply and home care resource consumption measures (Benjamin, 1986), but higher hospital discharge rates and shorter lengths of hospital stay have been associated with a greater prevalence of home care use in the Medicare population (Kenney & Dubay, 1992). Finally, Cohen and Tumlinson (1997) found that Medicare home care use at the state level was higher in states that had more restrictive Medicaid budgets, fewer Medicaid home care options, and fewer nursing home beds. This study provided the strongest evidence to date of cost shifting from Medicaid to Medicare in the home care arena.

HOME CARE RESOURCE CONSUMPTION AND PATIENT OUTCOMES

Thus far, we have discussed criteria that allow patients to consume home care resources, alternative ways of measuring home care resource consumption by eligible patients, and factors that are associated with level of resource consumption. In this section, we turn to the question of how patient outcomes are associated with resource consumption. In other words, how do patients fare as a result of receiving varying amounts of nursing, therapy, and paraprofessional services in their homes? Research evidence suggests that home care patient outcomes may be adversely affected by managed care arrangements, where pressures to reduce visits and to downgrade staffing levels are more prevalent (Shaughnessy, Schlenker, & Hittle, 1994; see also chapter 8). However, empirical relationships between resource consumption measures and patient outcome measures are not well understood, especially over episodes of home care.

To address this knowledge gap, a recent study examined how home care resource consumption patterns are associated with two patient outcome measures—discharge disposition at the end of a home care episode, and change in clinical and functional health status over the home care episode (Fortinsky & Madigan, 1997). This prospective cohort study included 201 patients from 10 Medicare-certified home care agencies in Ohio. The approach used by Shaughnessy and colleagues (1994) to define an episode of care was adopted for this study.

Discharge disposition categories were hospitalized, remained at home, and continued receiving home care beyond 62 days. Pain level and amount of dyspnea were used as clinical health status measures. Ability to perform four ADLs—ambulation, bathing, transferring, and grooming—were used as functional health status measures. For each health status measure, admission and discharge values were compared to obtain a change measure over the episode of home care. Patients were then classified as declined, remained stable, or improved from admission to discharge. Resource consumption was measured as the total number of home visits made by all disciplines during the study episode.

Results revealed that patients receiving home care beyond 62 days were much greater consumers of home care resources during the 62-day study period than either patients discharged home or those discharged to hospitals. Mean total numbers of home visits for these three patient groups were 26.3, 15.2, and 14.0, respectively ($p < .001$). Hospitalized patients consumed home care resources equivalent to those for patients who remained home, but in roughly half the amount of time; mean episode lengths were 18 days for hospitalized patients and 33 days for patients who remained at home. The study also showed that there were no statistically significant relationships between health status outcome measures and total number of visits. In other words, resource consumption patterns were very similar regardless of whether patients improved or declined in clinical and functional health during the episode of home care (Fortinsky & Madigan, 1997).

These study results suggest that relationships between home care resource consumption and patient outcomes are quite complex. Greater resource consumption clearly does not always lead to better outcomes, and indeed is as likely to lead to poorer outcomes. One explanation for these results is that home care staff may be initially deployed with the aim of achieving health improvement, but patients may decline in health during the home care episode, leading to greater staff deployment to either reverse or stabilize the decline. Thus, home care providers may change their service-provision decisions based on patient changes during an episode of home care. Research strategies to capture such phenomena would involve standardized, concise approaches for capturing clinical and functional health status of patients at each visit during an episode, combined with standardized approaches for measuring provider decisions about subsequent staff deployment following those same visits. These provider and research perspectives should be pursued to learn more about how resource consumption and patient outcome patterns could be optimally aligned in future home care service delivery.

CONCLUSIONS AND UNANSWERED QUESTIONS

The four central issues that framed this chapter were (1) the impact of home care eligibility criteria, employed by government, on home care resource consumption; (2) strategies for measuring resource consumption in home care; (3) known predictors of home care resource consumption; and (4) how home care resource consumption is related to patient outcomes. What conclusions can be reached regarding each of these issues, and what unanswered questions continue to limit our knowledge about what drives home care resource consumption in the United States?

Regarding eligibility criteria, we have seen that terminology embedded in Medicare home care policy leaves ample room for variation in interpretation of criteria such as homebound and intermittent. Decisions made by Medicare's regional FIs and home care providers suggest a lack of uniform interpretation of eligibility criteria, although little systematic research has been conducted to verify widely cited anecdotes in this area. In Medicaid waiver programs recent evidence clearly indicates wide variation in eligibility criteria across the states (O'Keeffe, 1996). Thus, even before home care resources are consumed by patients, we know that access to such services is highly influenced by decision-making processes by regulators and providers that are not well understood.

Regarding the state of the art in measuring home care resource consumption, we focused on Medicare home care because of the rapid pace of events in Medicare home care policy. We found that the home care visit continues to serve as the standard of home care resource consumption, even under the current interim payment system enacted as part of the BBA97. However, BBA97 also requires the implementation of a Medicare home care prospective payment system by 2001. Most likely, this new payment system will be based on episodes of care rather than visits, which may influence home care agency decisions about the length of visits to maximize productivity within episodes of care. Therefore, it appears that length of the visit and the home care episode will assume greater importance under new Medicare systems of payment and, concomitantly, also become more salient measures in research on resource consumption patterns. In addition, we contend that research on changes and variations in staff mix patterns over episodes of care will enhance our understanding of home care resource consumption patterns under prospective payment systems.

With respect to known predictors of resource consumption, the home care research literature clearly provides strong evidence of the influence of patient factors — especially health-related "need" factors at admission to home care—on resource consumption (measured primarily as number of visits). A study using national home care data examined the interplay between patient and agency factors and showed higher levels of resource consumption by proprietary agencies, compared to not-for-profit and governmental agencies, even after controlling for patient factors (Madigan, 1996). This study supports findings from smaller-scale studies (Ballard & McNamara, 1983; Edwardson & Nardone, 1991), and suggests the potentially important influence of decision-making processes occurring within home care agencies in affecting levels of resource consumption.

Regarding relationships between home care resource consumption and patient outcomes, recent work (Fortinsky & Madigan, 1997) strongly suggests that much more research is needed to understand the optimal numbers of visits needed to achieve beneficial outcomes. Decisions made by providers based only on patient need at admission could be detrimental to patient outcomes, since it is not clear how many visits patients need to attain maximum benefit. Much more needs to be learned about decisions made by home care clinicians and administrators once an episode of home care has begun, particularly as patients' conditions improve or worsen over the course of an episode.

Additional Questions

In considering causes and consequences of home care resource consumption in the future, there are three additional questions that should be addressed. First, how will patterns of home care resource consumption and patient outcomes be affected by managed care arrangements, especially under Medicare? Second, to what extent should home care consumers (patients and families) be involved in the home care decision making process? Finally, to what extent will the distinction between postacute and long-term home care be sustained for the growing population of patients with acute exacerbations of multiple chronic illnesses?

It is too early to know how the various managed care mechanisms under study will influence either home care resource consumption or patient outcomes. Some evidence suggests that home care patients who receive care from fee-for-service agencies consume more resources, but attain better outcomes, than those who receive care from HMO agencies (Shaughnessy et al., 1994). Another study, however, has found preliminary evidence that cost-reimbursed HMO home care does not differ from fee-for-service care in terms of resource consumption (Adams & Kramer, 1996). Preliminary research based on a wider array of health services suggests that chronically ill and poor and elderly persons fare worse under an HMO service environment than under the fee-for-service environment (Ware, Bayliss, Rogers, Kosinski, & Tarlov, 1996).

Numerous complicated issues cloud the arena of home care in a managed care era. One issue is whether home care agencies share in the financial risk arrangement (e.g., receive capitated payments), or whether they are paid in a cost-based manner by another group that holds the risk. Another issue is the degree of horizontal and vertical integration in the health system of which home agencies are a part. A third issue concerns the amount of managed care penetration in diverse geographic areas where home care agencies are located. All of these issues represent variables that could influence how much decision-making control agencies have as managed care opportunities are translated into resource consumption patterns and, ultimately, patient outcomes.

Related to the managed care question is the issue of who should decide on the level of home care resource consumption. Although there has been some movement toward involving patients and their family caregivers in decisions about long-term home care services (Riley, Fortinsky, & Coburn, 1992), no such movement is evident in Medicare home care, possibly because skilled care is assumed to be too clinically sophisticated for consumers to understand. However, little is known about how knowledgeable Medicare home care patients or their families may be about their health conditions, particularly in the sense of helping home care nurses decide which types of staff might assist in patients' recovery from acute exacerbations of chronic illnesses. Greater consumer involvement in Medicare home care decision-making may have the added advantage of sensitizing consumers to the realities of balancing resource availability with optimization of patient outcomes.

Finally, it is not clear how long the historic distinction between Medicare (postacute home care) vs. Medicaid and other public funding for long-term home care will remain viable. A growing number of states are actively pursuing strategies to pool Medicare and Medicaid funds to help integrate services for persons eligible for both public programs, known as dual-eligibles (Rosenbach & Lamphere, 1999). When combined with capitated payments for patients, such pooled funding systems may completely eliminate the distinction between postacute and long-term home care for poor older persons. Such pooling schemes would also reduce incentives to leverage Medicare dollars to replace state Medicaid and other public funding sources to pay for home care (Cohen & Tumlinson, 1997). Under less progressive financing scenarios, if more Medicare managed care pressures yield fewer visits and shorter lengths of stay in Medicare home care, will the long-term home care system be able to fill the remaining service needs of patients? In other words, changes to the Medicare home care system will have "downstream" effects in the long-term care system, so that any cost savings realized in Medicare programs may be shifted to nursing facilities if long-term home care cannot fill the service gap. Therefore, we would urge caution in home care planning to be sure that the policy changes do not result in shifts to higher cost providers.

In conclusion, while there is much activity in response to home care resource consumption trends, there is still much to learn about how decisions are and should be made to maximize the cost-effectiveness of home care in the United States. We urge greater collaboration at state and local levels between decision-makers contemplating changes in Medicare home care and those responsible for policy decisions affecting Medicaid and other publicly funded long-term home. We also encourage further research that includes a mix of qualitative and quantitative methods to improve our understanding about what factors drive decisions about resource consumption in addition to considerations of patient need for services at admission to an episode of home care. This type of research will help to shed light on the rapidly evolving home care arena.

REFERENCES

Adams, C. E., & Kramer, S. (1996). Home health resource utilization: Health maintenance organization versus fee-for-service subscribers. *Journal of Nursing Administration, 26,* 20–27.

Andersen, R. M. (1995). Revisiting the behavioral model and access to medical care: Does it matter? *Journal of Health and Social Behavior, 36,* 1–10.

Andersen, R. M., & Newman, J. F. (1973). Societal and individual determinants of medical care utilization in the United States. *Milbank Memorial Fund Quarterly, 51*(1), 91–124.

Ballard, S., & McNamara, R. (1983). Quantifying nursing needs in home health care. *Nursing Research, 32,* 236–241.

Benjamin, A. E. (1986). Determinants of state variation in home health utilization and expenditures under Medicare. *Medical Care, 24,* 535–547.

Bishop, C. E., Brown, R. S., Phillips, B., Ritter, G., & Skwara, K. C. (1996). The home health visit: An appropriate unit for Medicare payment? *Health Affairs, 15*(4), 145–155.

Branch, L. G., & Goldberg, H. B. (1993). A preliminary case mix classification system for Medicare home health clients. *Medical Care, 31,* 309–321.

Branch L. G., Goldberg, H. B., Cheh, V. A., & Williams, J. (1993). Medicare home health: A description of total episodes of care. *Health Care Financing Review, 14*(4), 59–74.

Branch, L., Jette, A., Evashwick, C., Polansky, M., Rowe, G., & Diehr, P. (1981). Toward understanding elders' health service utilization. *Journal of Community Health, 7,* 80–92.

Branch, L., Wetle, T. T., Scherr, P. A., Cook, N. R., Evans, D. A., Hebert, L. E., Masland, E. N., Keough, M. E., & Taylor, J. O. (1988). A prospective study of incident comprehensive medical home care use among the elderly. *American Journal of Public Health, 78,* 255–259.

Clauser, S. B. (1994). Recent innovations in home health care policy research. *Health Care Financing Review, 16*(1), 1–6.

Cohen, M. A., & Tumlinson, A. (1997). Understanding the state variation in Medicare home health care. *Medical Care, 35,* 618–633.

Coleman, B. (1999). *Trends in Medicaid long-term care spending* (Data Digest No. 38). Washington, D. C: American Association of Retired Persons, Public Policy Institute.

Coughlin, T. A., McBride, T. D., Perozek, M., & Liu, K. (1992). Home care for the disabled elderly: Predictors and expected costs. *Health Services Research, 27,* 453–479.

DiMaggio, P. J., & Powell, W. W. (1983). The iron cage revisited: Institutional isomorphism and collective rationality in organization fields. *American Sociological Review, 82,* 147–160.

Edwardson, S. R., & Nardone, P. (1991). Resource use in home care agencies. *Applied Nursing Research, 4,* 25–30.

Estes, C. L., & Swan, J. H. (1994). Privatization, system membership, and access to home health care for the elderly. *Milbank Quarterly, 72,* 277–298.

Evashwick, C., Rowe, G., Diehr, P., & Branch, L. (1984). Factors explaining the use of health care services by the elderly. *Health Services Research, 19,* 357–382.

Fortinsky, R. H., Hathaway, T. J., & McGuire, C. (1992). *Evaluation of publicly funded home care services for older adults in Maine.* Portland, ME: Muskie Institute of Public Affairs, University of Southern Maine.

Fortinsky, R. H., & Madigan, E. A. (1997). Home care resource consumption and patient outcomes: What are the relationships? *Home Health Care Services Quarterly, 16*(3), 55–73.

Gage, B., Stevenson, D., Liu, K., & Aragon, C. (1998). Medicare home health: An update. *Public Policy and Aging Report, 9,* 12–15.

Goldberg, H. B. (1997). Personal communication, February 19.

Goldberg, H. B., & Schmitz, R. J. (1994). Contemplating home health PPS: Current patterns of Medicare service use. *Health Care Financing Review, 16*(1), 109–130.

Haupt, B. J. (1998). *An overview of home health and hospice care patients: 1996 National Home and Hospice Care Survey* (Advance Data from Vital and Health Statistics, No. 297). Hyattsville, MD: National Center for Health Statistics.

Health Care Financing Administration. (1998). *Medicare and Medicaid Statistical supplement, 1998. Health Care Financing Review.*

Hegner, R. E. (1996). *Medicare coverage for home health care: Reining in a benefit out of control.* (Issue Brief No. 694). Washington, DC: National Health Policy Forum.

Hoyer, R. G. (1995). Prospective payment for home care. *CARING, 14*(3), 28–36.

Ingoldsby, A. I., Kumar, N., Cohen, M. A., & Wallack, S. S. (1994). Medicare home health care: The struggle for definition. *Journal of Long-Term Home Health Care, 13*(3), 16–31.

Kane, R. L., Finch, M., Chen, Q., Blewett, L., Burns, R., & Moskowitz, M. (1994). Post-hospital home health care for Medicare patients. *Health Care Financing Review, 16*(1), 131–153.

Kemper, P. (1992). The use of formal and informal care by the disabled elderly. *Health Services Research, 27,* 421–451.

Kenney, G. M., & Dubay, L. C. (1992). Explaining area variation in the use of Medicare home health services. *Medical Care, 30,* 43–57.

Kenney, G., & Moon, M. (1997). *Reining in the growth in home health services under Medicare.* Washington, DC: The Urban Institute.

Levit, K. R., Lazenby, H. C., Braden, B. R., Cowan, C. A., Sensenig, A. L., McDonnell, P. A., Stiller, J. M., Won, D. K., Martin, A. B., Sivarajan, L., Donham, C. S., Long, A. M., & Stewart, M. W. (1997). National health expenditures 1996. *Health Care Financing Review, 19*(1), 161–200.

Madigan, E. A. (1996). *Determinants of service provision in home care agencies, 1992.* Unpublished doctoral dissertation. Case Western Reserve University, Cleveland.

Madigan, E. A., & Fortinsky, R. H. (1999). Alternative measures of resource consumption in home care episodes. *Public Health Nursing, 16,* 198–204.

Mauser, E. (1997). Medicare home health initiative: Current activities and future directions. *Health Care Financing Review, 18*(3), 275–291.

McAuley, W. J., & Arling, G. (1984). Use of in-home care by very old people. *Journal of Health and Social Behavior, 25,* 54–64.

National Association for Home Care. (1997). *Transition to PPS: The interim payment system for Medicare home health services.* Washington, DC: Author.

O'Keeffe, J. (1996). *Determining the need for long-term care services: An analysis of health and functional eligibility criteria in Medicaid home and community-based waiver programs.* Washington, DC: American Association of Retired Persons, Public Policy Institute.

Pasquale, D. K. (1987). A basis for prospective payment for home care. *Image: Journal of Nursing Scholarship, 19,* 186–191.

Payne, S. M. C., Thomas, C. P., Fitzpatrick, T., Abdel-Rahman, M., & Kayne, H. L. (1998). Determinants of home health visit length: Results of a multisite prospective study. *Medical Care, 36,* 1500–1514.

Pettigrew, M. L., Kramer, A. M., & Shaughnessy, P. W. (1988). Hospital-based and freestanding home health case mix: Implications for Medicare reimbursement policy. *Home Health Care Services Quarterly, 8,* 75–88.

Phillips, B. R., Brown, R. S., & Bishop, C. E. (1994). Do preset per visit payment rates affect home health agency behavior? *Health Care Financing Review, 16*(1), 91–107.

Riley, P., Fortinsky, R. H., & Coburn, A. F. (1992). Developing consumer-centered quality assurance strategies for home care: A case management model. *Journal of Case Management, 1,* 39–48.

Rosenbach, M. L., & Lamphere, J. (1999). *Bridging the gaps between Medicare and Medicaid: The case of QMBs and SLMBs* (Publication No. 9902). Washington, DC: American Association for Retired Persons, Public Policy Institute.

Schlenker, R. E. (1996). *Home health payment legislation: Review and recommendations.* Washington, DC: American Association of Retired Persons, Public Policy Institute.

Schore, J. (1996). *Regional variation in Medicare home health. Taking a closer look.* Princeton, NJ: Mathematica Policy Research.

Shaughnessy, P. W., Crisler, K. S., Schlenker, R. E., Arnold, A. G., Kramer, A. M., Powell, M. C., & Hittle, D. F. (1994). Measuring and assuring the quality of home health care. *Health Care Financing Review, 16*(1), 35–67.

Shaughnessy, P. W., Schlenker, R. E., & Hittle, D. F. (1994). Home health care outcomes under capitated and fee-for-service payment. *Health Care Financing Review, 16*(1), 187–222.

Shuster, G. F., & Cloonan, P. A. (1991). Home health nursing care: A comparison of not-for-profit and for-profit agencies. *Home Health Care Services Quarterly, 12,* 23–36.

Soldo, B. J. (1985). In-home services for the dependent elderly. *Research on Aging, 7,* 281–304.

Solomon, D. H., Wagner, R., Maremberg, M. E., Acampora, D., Cooney, L. M., & Iouye, S. K. (1993). Predictors of formal home health care use in elderly patients after hospitalization. *Journal of the American Geriatrics Society, 41,* 961–966.

Starrett, R. A., Rogers, D., & Walters, G. (1989). Home health care utilization: A causal model. *Home Health Care Services Quarterly, 9,* 125–140.

Swan, J. H. & Benjamin, A. E. (1993). Nursing home queues and home health users. *Home Health Care Services Quarterly, 14*(4), 157–173.

Swan, J. H., Black, L., Benjamin, A. E., & Fox, P. (1995). Use of covered services in Medicare home health care. *Home Health Care Services Quarterly, 15*(4), 1–18.

Ware, J. E., Bayliss, M. S., Rogers, W. H., Kosinski, M., & Tarlov, A. R. (1996). Differences in 4–year health outcomes for elderly and poor, chronically ill patients treated in HMO and fee-for-service systems: Results from the Medical Outcomes Study. *Journal of the American Medical Association, 276,* 1039–1047.

Welch, H. G., Wennberg, D. E., & Welch, W. P. (1996). The use of Medicare home health care services. *New England Journal of Medicine, 335,* 324–329.

Williams, B. (1994). Comparison of services among different types of home health agencies. *Medical Care, 32,* 1134–1152.

CHAPTER 8

Shaping Home Care by Measuring Outcomes

Peter W. Shaughnessy

The nature and extent of home care are being shaped by demographics and consumer preference as well as substantial changes in Medicare, Medicaid, managed care, and home care itself. This confluence of evolving trends has produced a platform for change that is anchored by four questions.

First, do Medicare and Medicaid spend too much on home care? The increase in utilization and cost of home care between 1988 and 1996 is virtually unprecedented in the history of the U.S. health care system (see

---

The research that forms the foundation for this paper was funded under several grants and contracts from different funding agencies; Health Care Financing Administration, HHS Cooperative Agreement No. 17-C-99051/8, and Contract Nos. 500-88-0054 and 500-94-0054; Agency for Health Care Policy and Research, HHS Grant No. 5 RO1 HS08031; Robert Wood Johnson Foundation Grant Nos. 13779 and 19218; a developmental grant from the National Association for Home Care; and Assistant Secretary for Planning and Evaluation, HHS Contract No. HHS-100-95-045.

Portions of this paper are also published in *Handbook of Home Health Care Administration* (2nd ed.), edited by Marilyn D. Harris. Gaithersburg, MD: Aspen Publishers, 1997.

chapter 1). Whether this growth is warranted and whether the cost of home care offsets or reduces costs of other types of health care are largely unknown. Prospective payment for home care providers, and managed care are viewed as means to control the cost and perhaps the growth of home care services (Schlenker, 1996). Yet, whether clients or patients benefit differentially from varying amounts of home care services and visits is unknown. We are unclear whether lower volume thresholds exist below which patient outcomes are markedly inferior, and whether upper thresholds exist above which there are no or diminishing returns in terms of patient outcomes. In considering this first question of whether Medicare and Medicaid spend excessively on home care, the bottom line is necessarily focused on both the outcomes and cost of home care.

The second general question raised by the confluence of the forces noted above deals with the cost effectiveness of home care. Closely related to the question of whether Medicare and Medicaid overspend on home care is the question of whether home care is cost effective. The optimal way to measure effectiveness is through outcomes. The (ideal) perspective that should be taken by a payer is that of a purchaser of enhanced health (outcomes), not simply a purchaser of care or services. Analogously, the (ideal) provider perspective is that of a producer of enhanced health (outcomes), not simply a provider of care or services. A fundamental question related to cost effectiveness is therefore what outcomes are purchased and produced at what cost? Again, the bottom line focuses on outcomes and cost.

In view of current trends in our health care system, the third question concerns the potential of Medicare and Medicaid as well as other types of managed care to control costs and constructively shape the pervasive growth of home care in the United States. The predominant users of home care, Medicare and Medicaid beneficiaries, are being encouraged to enroll in managed care plans at unprecedented rates. What do we know about managed care relative to home care? Is home care less costly under managed care? Is it as effective? Over the course of time, will managed care function more efficiently as those who administer and direct managed care organizations learn more about how to purchase enhanced outcomes? In this context, as above, the bottom line is apparent and again involves the outcomes and costs of home care—in this case, under managed care payment environments.

The fourth question is, What should we do to shape, guide, and channel the growth of home care? What should be our game plan or vision? Can we specify a target? Or, can we at least specify a vehicle to help us learn more about the growth and nature of home care in order to facilitate our ability to articulate a target? In doing so, an elemental response to this question, in view of the foregoing points on outcomes and cost, is that in our thinking, in our monitoring, in our actions, and in paying for and providing home care, considerations regarding cost and patient/client outcomes must converge. How can we bring this convergence about? What kinds of information should we collect and monitor to do so?

This chapter presents research that has been undertaken to help answer these questions. It begins with an account of a study that demonstrates how such research can compare a number of dimensions of home health care delivered by HMOs with care provided under the fee-for-service payment system. Next, it explicates a system of outcome measures that have been developed and utilized for measuring quality of care. Then, it demonstrates how measures of outcomes and costs of care can be integrated. It concludes with a discussion of future development and refinement of methods to measure home care outcomes and resource consumption.

IS MANAGED CARE THE ANSWER? AN ILLUSTRATION

The increased provision of home care through managed care auspices provides an arena for illustrating one way in which outcome measures can be usefully applied. By design, at least on conceptual grounds, the purpose of managed care is to maintain health by determining health care needs of a given individual or a population (of enrollees) and thereafter make the most efficient use of the entire spectrum of health services, to prevent, ameliorate, or resolve health problems that might be due to either natural progression of disease or iatrogenic factors (Birnbaum, 1976; Morrison & Luft, 1990). Managed care should facilitate efficient and effective patient-level transitions from one provider setting to another (Christianson, 1980; Enthoven & Kronick, 1989a, 1989b). This would ideally result from focusing on the entire patient and from monitoring health status over time and across provider settings. Because of this orientation, we would expect managed care organizations to have a strong interest in measuring and monitoring outcomes over specific episodes of care as well as over longer intervals of time that span multiple care episodes. To assess the cost and outcomes of home care under managed care (HMOs in particular), a comparative study of cost, quality, case mix, and utilization of Medicare home health care under HMOs versus fee-for-service (FFS) payment was undertaken by the University of Colorado's Center for Health Services Research.

Three types of home health agencies were included in the study. HMO-owned agencies are totally owned and managed by HMOs. The study included 9 such agencies and 308 patients from these agencies. The second type of agency is pure-FFS agencies, which do virtually no business with HMOs (less than 2% of total admissions from HMOs for study agencies). Fifteen pure-FFS agencies were included in this study, with 529 patients from these agencies. The third type consists of contractual agencies that do a substantial HMO and FFS business (contractual agencies were defined to have at least 15 HMO admissions and 15 FFS admissions per month). The study included 14 contractual agencies, with 381 HMO patients and 414 FFS patients from these agencies. The study agencies were Medicare certified, and all managed care plans were TEFRA-risk HMOs.* Patients for whom primary data were collected were Medicare patients 65 years of age or older. Longitudinal data were collected on site at admission and every 3 weeks thereafter until and including time of discharge. Patients were followed for 12 weeks or until discharge, whichever occurred first. Data were collected at each time point for individual patients and included over 200 items per patient on physiologic, functional, cognitive, and behavioral indicators of health status. Information also was collected on home environment, demographics, service provision, and resource consumption.

More comprehensive results and the methodology for the study are published elsewhere (Schlenker, Shaughnessy, & Hittle, 1995; Shaughnessy, Schlenker, & Hittle, 1994, 1995). Selected findings and implications of the study are highlighted here to serve the more general purposes of this chapter. Cost and outcome findings are summarized, with additional details as well as case mix and utilization results available in the references noted.

Figure 8.1 contains the 12–week cost findings pertaining to agency-incurred personnel costs of providing home care to patients over the 12–week-or-discharge interval. On the left side are the overall HMO versus

---

*The Tax Equity and Fiscal Responsibility Act (TEFRA, P. L. 97-248) of 1982 provided the enabling legislation for Medicare to contract with HMOs on a risk basis.

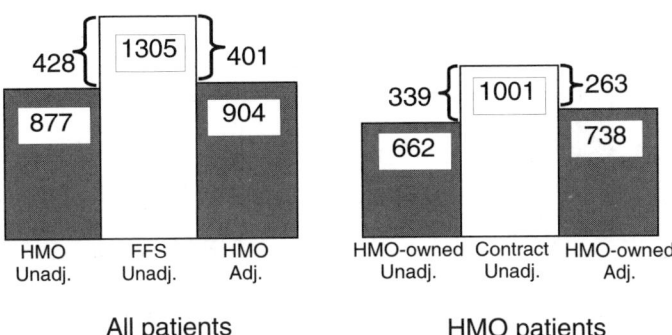

FIGURE 8.1. Illustrative HMO versus FFS patient-level cost findings adjusted for case mix, demographics, agency, and regional covariates.*
*Adjusted costs are based on regression analyses.

FFS findings. For all FFS patients pooled (i.e., FFS patients from both pure-FFS and contractual agencies), the average cost over the study interval was $1,305. The analogous cost for all HMO patients (HMO patients from both HMO-owned and contractual agencies) was $877, less than the FFS average cost by $428. After adjusting for case mix, demographics, agency, and regional covariates, this difference was reduced to $401 ($p < .01$). Analogous case mix–adjusted cost differences were found between FFS and HMO payment environments within the contractual pool of patients and within the pool of patients from HMO-owned and pure-FFS agencies. The results on the right side of Figure 8.1 indicate that home care provided to HMO patients receiving care from contractual agencies was more costly than the home care provided to patients receiving care from HMO-owned agencies. This was contrary to our original hypothesis, which specified HMO-owned home health agencies would be likely to use home care services more creatively and extensively to avoid hospitalization and other expensive types of care because more extensive use of home care services would tend to increase visits and therefore personnel costs.

From the vantage point of cost alone, these findings suggest that an HMO or managed care payment environment is superior to a fee-for-service payment environment. In view of the aforementioned bottom line

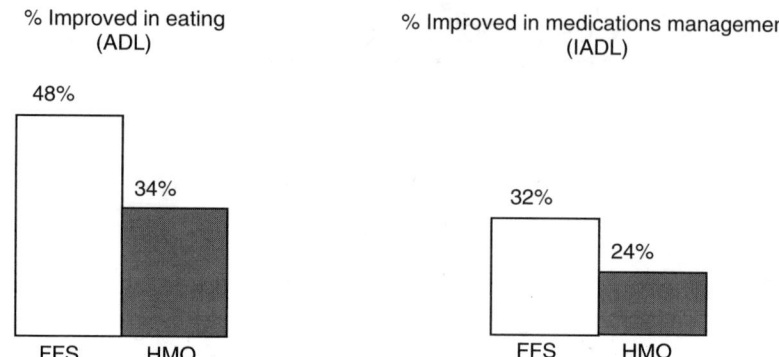

FIGURE 8.2. Illustrative HMO versus FFS patient-level risk-adjusted outcome findings at 12 weeks or discharge, whichever occurred first, for improvement in eating and improvement in medications management.

that should focus on both costs and outcomes, the results also raise the question of outcomes, or what happens to patients.

As with the cost findings that highlight the general pattern of results, the outcome findings in Figure 8.2 are illustrative of a general set of outcome findings. These results pertain to pooled-HMO versus pooled-FFS patients (as do the cost results on the left side of Figure 8.1). The risk-adjusted outcome findings based on logistic regression models indicate that the outcome of "improved in eating" (an activity of daily living [ADL]) was 14 percentage points (or 41%) higher for FFS patients. Analogously, the result on the right side of Figure 8.2 demonstrates that the risk-adjusted outcome of "improved in medications management" (an instrumental activity of daily living [IADL]) was 8 percentage points (or 33%) higher for FFS patients relative to HMO patients. Both differences in Figure 8.2 are statistically significant ($p < .10$).

The results in Figure 8.3 further illustrate the nature of the outcome findings for FFS versus HMO patients. The risk-adjusted results in this figure indicate that stabilization in transferring and stabilization in an aggregate indicator of ADL disabilities (including the ADLs of bathing, grooming, eating, toileting, and transferring) were significantly superior for FFS patients ($p < .005$). The overall set of findings showed that of the 55 outcome measures used, 14 yielded statistically significant differences after risk adjustment, with all such differences reflecting inferior outcomes for HMO patients (Shaughnessy, Schlenker, & Hittle, et al., 1994).

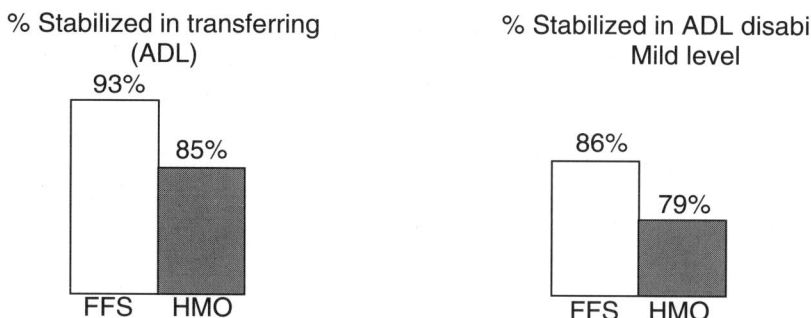

FIGURE 8.3. Illustrative HMO versus FFS patient-level risk-adjusted outcome findings at 12 weeks or discharge, whichever occurred first, stabilized in transferring and stabilized in mild disabilities in aggregate ADL index.

Applying a nonparametric (sign) test to all outcome measure differences demonstrated that a significantly greater portion of all health status outcome measures (49 of 55) were superior for FFS patients.

The general superiority of outcomes for FFS patients persisted when comparing HMO patients admitted to HMO-owned agencies with FFS patients admitted to pure-FFS agencies, and when comparing contractual HMO patients with contractual FFS patients. The nature of the outcome differences for these two comparative analyses was slightly different than for the pooled comparisons indicated above, but the overall pattern of superior outcomes for FFS patients tended to persist (with some exceptions). Further details on precisely how the measures were computed, the nature of the risk adjustment, statistical significance associated with the comparisons of all outcome measures, and results of nonparametric tests are given in the references cited above.

From a policy perspective, the results of this study of HMO and FFS patients receiving home care suggest that we should have concern about the quality of home health care provided under HMO auspices. In this regard, qualifications of these findings are given in other publications (see references noted above), but one should be noted here. It is possible that, after a period of approximately 6 months (i.e., beyond the 12–week study interval), outcomes for HMO patients might be the same as the outcomes for FFS patients. That is, the provision of more frequent and possibly superior home care services to FFS patients may simply accelerate attaining outcomes that eventually reach the same level at a later time with other types of ambulatory care provided by HMOs. However, because several of the types of patients monitored had rehabilitation conditions (e.g., poststroke), it is unlikely that this "catch up" would occur for all patients because there is some clinical evidence in support of the permanent beneficial impacts of rehabilitation provided immediately after certain traumatic events (Granger & Clark, 1994; Granger & Hamilton, 1990; Granger et al., 1996; Greenspun, 1994). Also, attaining outcomes more quickly can be beneficial to patients in several ways, such as increased work productivity, quality of life, and avoidance of complications. Nonetheless, because these findings pertain to only a 12–week interval, there is some room to challenge them. Thus, the results suggest, but do not necessarily prove, that the higher home care costs for FFS patients are offset (or possibly more than offset) by the higher levels of positive outcomes for these patients. Regardless, the approach demonstrates one method for comparing costs and outcomes concurrently—that is, addressing the combined bottom line mentioned earlier. Furthermore, the methodology points to the value of monitoring patient outcomes, a topic that will now be discussed in more detail.

MONITORING OUTCOMES

The study comparing costs and outcomes in HMO and FFS home care, just summarized, is one of a series of activities undertaken by the Center for Health Services Research, University of Colorado Health Sciences Center, that have provided opportunities to test and refine quality measures under various circumstances. Over the past 15 years we have been developing a system of quality measures for home care and, to some extent, for long-term care in general.

The purpose of the center's program is to develop quality measures, largely outcome measures, premised on the assumption that providers of care, regulators, payers, consumers, and managed care organizations should be familiar with, challenged by, and make extensive use of information on what happens to patients and clients as a result of receiving home care services. At the same time, we cannot be unrealistic in attempting to employ excessively broad-based measures of quality of life to assure quality of care, because so many exogenous circumstances influence quality of life (including prior choices by consumers and their families, as well as an exceptionally wide array of risk factors). Therefore, we must be judicious in selecting realistic and useful measures for continuous quality improvement (CQI), including practical ones that reflect quality of life. Not to be ignored in this regard is the importance of functioning reflected by both ADLs and IADLs. For individuals to remain at home, functioning at some level is essential (depending on the nature and extent of the home support system). Because of this and the fact that functioning, broadly defined, is a necessary condition for independence, for participating in a range of activities, and for accomplishing a variety of objectives, functional outcomes can be regarded as important in the context of measuring quality of life.* The measure system that has evolved over the past several years presently is based on an array of functional and physiologic measures as well as selected cognitive, social, and mental health outcome measures.

The evolution of the outcome measure system and the quality improvement approach based on this measure system, termed outcome-based quality improvement (OBQI), has involved a number of separate but integrated activities (Shaughnessy, 1991; Shaughnessy, Crisler, Schlenker, & Arnold, 1995; Shaughnessy, Crisler, et al., 1994; Shaughnessy, Schlenker, et al., 1996). These have included comprehensive reviews of outcome measures and related papers, documents, and articles published in research literature and the provider and clinical literature, as well as reviews of outcome measures in use or under development by individual agencies or groups of agencies. A number of clinical panels have been convened to review the outcome measures and approaches at regular intervals over time. A variety of different data sources were examined for potential information on outcome measurement. Outcome measures were specified first, and data items needed to measure outcomes were developed thereafter. Extant sources of information for such data items were examined, including clinical records, claims or billing data, and other administrative data. After an extensive examination of such data sources, we concluded it would be necessary to develop a new data set to properly measure the outcomes that had been specified. Several hundred home care agencies throughout the United States participated in the de-

---

*Also related to quality of life is the importance of consumer/family/caregiver volitional measures that reflect patient choice, and the opportunity to control the type of care and care environment. As implied earlier, while measuring health outcomes across a spectrum of domains of health bears promise, we should exercise caution in using expansive quality of life measures that have not yet been shown to be practical for quality improvement.

velopmental efforts over a period of several years, including various types of research investigations, data item refinement (including validity and reliability testing), and both demonstration and evaluation projects (Crisler et al., 1994; Powell et al., 1994; Shaughnessy, Crisler, Schlenker, & Arnold, 1995; Shaughnessy, Crisler, et al., 1994; Shaughnessy, Schlenker, et al., 1994).

The resulting and still evolving system is currently under consideration by the Health Care Financing Administration (HCFA) for national implementation in the context of its Medicare Survey and Certification Program for home health agencies. The overall plan is to incorporate outcomes into the certification process, so that agencies that are performing adequately or above average in terms of outcomes will receive relatively little survey/certification/regulatory review, with such review focusing predominantly on agencies for whom outcomes are inadequate. For the latter agencies, regulatory activities can be targeted on those areas where outcomes are inferior. The system described here is therefore intended for application by individual home health agencies and by purchasers of care who wish to assess what is happening to patients/clients as a result of their financial investment in home care. (This description provides an overview of the basic features of the OBQI approach as they were developed prior to the mid-1990s. Changes and refinements occurring thereafter will continue to be published and can be obtained by contacting the author or the Center for Health Services Research, University of Colorado Health Sciences Center. Further details on the types of measures, overall system, and plans for the future are available through the sources cited above.)

Types of Outcomes

The fundamental definition of a patient-level outcome is a change in health status between two or more time points. In the current OBQI system, this is the basic or anchoring definition of an outcome. It is termed an end-result outcome because it reflects change in patient health over the course of time, which is the focal point of health care. The two time points that are typically used to gauge outcomes in home care are start of care (SOC) and discharge. Health status, as noted above, is broadly defined, encompassing physiologic, functional, cognitive, mental, and social health. Illustrations of end-result outcomes include improvement in ability to ambulate between admission and discharge, improvement in ability to manage oral medications between admission and discharge, decline in dyspnea between admission and 120 days after admission, and stabilization or no change in pain interfering with activities between 60 and 180 days. The third and fourth illustrations demonstrate that it is not necessary to consider SOC and discharge as the only two follow-up points that define outcomes.

A second type of outcome used that is under development for future use in OBQI is termed an instrumental outcome (or intermediate-result outcome). An instrumental outcome is a change in patient (or informal caregiver's) behavior, emotions, or knowledge that can influence a patient's end-result outcomes. Illustrations of instrumental outcomes include change in compliance with treatment regimen, knowledge of self-care, knowledge of signs and symptoms to report, informal caregiver strain, patient or family satisfaction with care, and motivation to improve. These are termed instrumental outcomes because, although outcomes in their own right, their (non)attainment can influence the (non)attainment of end-result outcomes. Instrumental outcomes are critical in home care but are more difficult to measure than end-result outcomes and therefore are not in widespread use in OBQI at the present time. However, it is anticipated that as additional research and developmental efforts focus on such outcomes, they will be used more widely in OBQI in the home care field.

The third type of outcomes is utilization outcomes, which refer to utilization of nonhome care services that reflects (typically a substantial and untoward) change in health status over time. Illustrations of utilization outcomes include hospital admission, nursing home admission, and emergent care. These are also termed proxy outcomes because they are often (but not always) surrogates for untoward or negative health status changes in patients. Such outcomes have the redeeming feature that they are more straightforward to measure, although risk adjustment is often of paramount importance in comparing such outcomes across different groups of patients.

Outcome Measures and Data Sets

An outcome measure is a quantification of an outcome. Under the assumption that the outcome under consideration is an end-result outcome, an outcome measure is a quantified change in patient health status between two or more time points. The change referred to in this case is intrinsic to the patient. (In contrast, provision of a cane or walker is not intrinsic to the patient and is therefore not an outcome). The change can represent improvement, stabilization, or worsening. Objective measures are superior to subjective measures. Thus, when quantifying outcomes, specific, reliable, and objective health status scales are preferable (for end-result and instrumental outcomes), and precise information on health care use is preferable to measure utilization outcomes.

A wide variety of outcomes and outcome measures were specified in the developmental research that underpins OBQI. Over time, these were culled, modified, or refined from different vantage points including clinical relevance, reliability, specificity, practicality, utility for QI purposes, and minimizing statistical redundancy. Efforts are ongoing to remedy various constraints and limitations of the system as well as to improve measures and develop new ones. Because the initial objectives focused on specifying outcome measures, all data items followed from the outcome measures. That is, OBQI data items were not first specified and then used to determine which measures would be possible. The primary focus was on outcome measures that could be integrated to form a system that would be valid and practical for OBQI, with all other considerations (including data items) secondary to this purpose.

The set of data items used in the OBQI system is termed the Outcome and ASsessment Information Set (OASIS). It was tailored to home care after investigating the appropriateness of using data items from other fields, such as the Functional Independence Measure (FIM) data set in the rehabilitation field and the Minimum Data Set (MDS) in the nursing home field (Fries et al., 1994; Granger, Hamilton, Linacre, Heineman, & Wright, 1993; Granger, Ottenbacher, & Fiedler, 1995; Hawes et al., 1995; Morris et al., 1990; State University of New York at Buffalo, 1993, 1995). Extensive modifications of these data sets would have been necessary to properly adapt them to home care; in addition, several of the items did not necessarily provide the information needed to measure the outcomes needed for home care.

The OASIS data set is continuing to undergo refinement, as is the scope of the OBQI home care measure system. The first release of the 79–item OASIS occurred in August 1995 as a special supplement to the National Association for Home Care's *NAHC Report* (National Association for Home Care, 1995). This was termed OASIS-A and is being followed by subsequent releases that will be termed OASIS-B, OASIS-C, etc. OASIS is not a comprehensive assessment instrument. Rather, it is a set of data items essential for measuring or risk adjusting outcomes in the home care field. It is strongly recommended that OASIS items be embedded within the comprehensive assessment instrument of each home care agency that uses the OBQI measure system. To simply add the OASIS items to an existing assessment instrument creates substantial redundancy, as almost all OASIS items have analogs in items that are already used for comprehensive assessment. To measure outcomes, it is necessary to collect OASIS data items at 60-day intervals until and including time of discharge. Further specifics are available in other research documents and the OBQI manual written for home care agencies wishing to implement OBQI (Shaughnessy & Crisler, 1995).

Implementing Outcome-based Quality Improvement

The general framework for OBQI is the two-stage CQI screen depicted in Figure 8.4. This schematic shows the overall OBQI approach. The sequence of events on the left side of Figure 8.4 constitutes the first-stage screen, and those on the right side constitute the second-stage screen. In order to conduct the two-stage CQI screen, data must be collected at the above-mentioned intervals for all adult patients. (The outcome measures pertain to adult patients, although the system will be expanded to pertain to other types of nonadult patients and specialized patients, such as terminal and short-stay patients that might be referred by managed care organizations.) The first-stage screen consists of out-

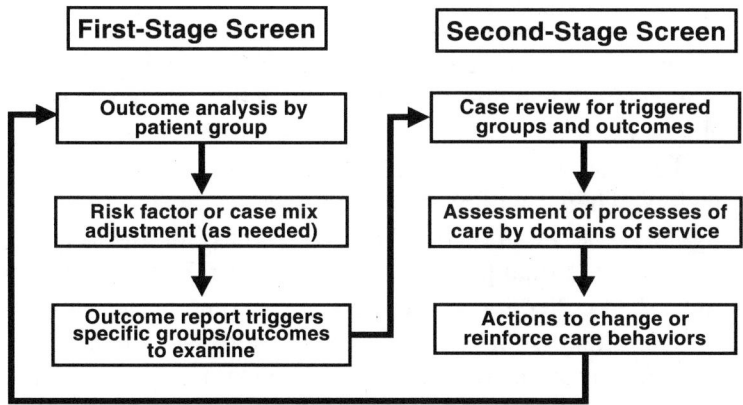

FIGURE 8.4. Two-stage continuous quality improvement screen.

come analyses by patient groups. This step entails computing outcome measures from the OBQI outcome measure system on a condition-by-condition basis, using quality indicator groups (QUIGs). Although there are a number of ways to stratify patients into groups, the QUIG classification system given in Table 8.1 has been developed for initial use and subsequent refinement for OBQI applications (Kramer, Shaughnessy, Bauman, & Crisler, 1990; Shaughnessy & Crisler, 1995). It consists of 25 (potentially overlapping) patient conditions for which outcome measures have been specified. After outcome measures are computed using the OASIS data set, risk adjustment is undertaken and outcome reports are produced for specific QUIGs of relevance to the agency (termed "focused" outcome reports) and for all adult patients (termed a "global" outcome report).

The production of outcome reports is the culmination of the first-stage screen. Using these reports (an illustration will be provided below), agency staff can then determine which outcomes are inferior and which are exemplary. The outcomes on which the agency staff elects to focus for purposes of subsequent review are called target outcomes and constitute the focal point of the second-stage screen. A variety of activities can be undertaken as part of the second-stage screen, but all activities deal with investigating care provided for purposes of reinforcing those care behaviors that produce exemplary outcomes, or with remedying problems in care behaviors that produce inferior outcomes. This usually entails record review for the triggered outcomes that correspond either to particular QUIGs or to all patients if the triggered outcomes are taken from a global outcome report. The review of services provided is often by domains of patient conditions and domains of services or processes of care.

The second-stage screen culminates with written plans of action specifically targeted at changing or reinforcing care behaviors that produce certain outcomes. A plan of action entails specifying what will be done, how it will be done, who will undertake the activities necessary to change care behaviors, when it will be done, and how the process of implementing change will be monitored. The effectiveness of the second-stage screen, including the final plans of action, can then be assessed by virtue of continued data collection and review of outcome reports for the next period of time. This permits agency staff to determine whether outcomes targeted for improvement have in fact improved and whether those targeted for reinforcement have remained the same or even improved. The heart of the CQI process, therefore, is producing outcome reports on a

TABLE 8.1 Description of Quality Indicator Groups (QUIGs) and Examples

Acute conditions

1. Acute orthopedic conditions (e.g., fracture, amputation, joint replacement, degenerative joint disease)
2. Acute neurologic conditions (e.g., cerebrovascular accident, multiple sclerosis, head injury)
3. Open wounds and lesions (e.g., pressure ulcers, surgical wounds, stasis ulcers)
4. Terminal conditions (e.g., palliative care for malignant neoplasms, advanced cardiopulmonary disease, end-stage AIDS)
5. Acute cardiac/peripheral vascular conditions (e.g., congestive heart failure, angina, coronary artery disease, hypertension, myocardial infarction)
6. Acute pulmonary conditions (e.g., chronic obstructive pulmonary disease, pneumonia, pulmonary edema)
7. Acute diabetes mellitus*
8. Acute gastrointestinal disorders (e.g., gastric ulcer, diverticulitis, constipation with changing treatment approaches, ostomies, liver disease)
9. Contagious/communicable conditions (e.g., hepatitis, tuberculosis, AIDS, salmonella)
10. Acute urinary incontinence/catheter*
11. Acute mental/emotional conditions (e.g., anxiety disorder, depression, bipolar disorder)
12. Oxygen therapy*
13. IV/Infusion therapy*
14. Enteral/parenteral nutrition (e.g., total parenteral nutrition, gastrostomy/jejunostomy feeding)
15. Ventilator therapy*
16. Other acute conditions*

Chronic conditions

17. Chronic dependence in living skills (e.g., meal preparation, housekeeping, laundry)
18. Chronic dependence in personal care (e.g., bathing, dressing, grooming)
19. Chronic impaired ambulation/mobility (e.g., ambulation, transferring, toileting)
20. Chronic eating disability*
21. Chronic urinary incontinence/catheter use*
22. Chronic dependence in medication administration*
23. Chronic pain*
24. Chronic cognitive/mental/behavioral problems (e.g., Alzheimer's, confusion, agitation, chronic brain syndrome)
25. Chronic patients with caregiver present*

*Example not given as QUIG name is sufficient to define condition.

regular basis that can be used to monitor outcomes of care and assess whether changes introduced to remedy inadequacies in care behaviors have improved outcomes and whether reinforcement activities implemented to maintain exemplary or superior outcomes have done so.

In the context of various demonstration programs, approximately 160 agencies are presently implementing and formally maintaining OBQI approaches that employ OASIS and the aforementioned system of outcome measures. In addition, a number of other home care agencies throughout the United States are beginning to implement OBQI under auspices of state associations, state governments, provider chains/corporations, provider coalitions, and even individual providers.

One of the more important OBQI demonstration projects is the national Medicare OBQI Demonstration program that is funded by HCFA. This large-scale test of the prototype OBQI system that will be used under Medicare involves 54 agencies from 26 states. It began in 1995 and will continue until 2001, with three rounds of data collection and outcome reporting. Outcome reports are being produced for the 54 participating agencies in late 1996, early 1998, and mid-1999. All agencies are collecting OASIS data for their nonmaternity adult home care patients. Outcome reports are risk adjusted, and the two-stage screen described previously is being implemented for each of the three rounds of outcome reports.

An analogous project was implemented in New York state in 1996. This project, involving 22 home care agencies from New York, will further test the OBQI system in terms of personal care and will entail at least two if not three rounds of data collection and outcome reporting before a final decision is made for statewide implementation in New York. A Colorado OBQI pilot project involving three agencies has been in place since 1992. (Further information on this pilot is presented below.) Also, because HCFA is planning to use OBQI in the context of its national quality assurance and improvement program, HCFA's per-episode prospective payment demonstration (involving 91 agencies from California, Texas, Illinois, Florida, and Massachusetts) is using OBQI to monitor and ensure the quality of home care (Abt Associates, 1995).

A Hypothetical Outcome Report

Figure 8.5 contains an excerpt from a hypothetical outcome report for an individual home care agency. It displays results for two improvement

Shaping Home Care by Measuring Outcomes

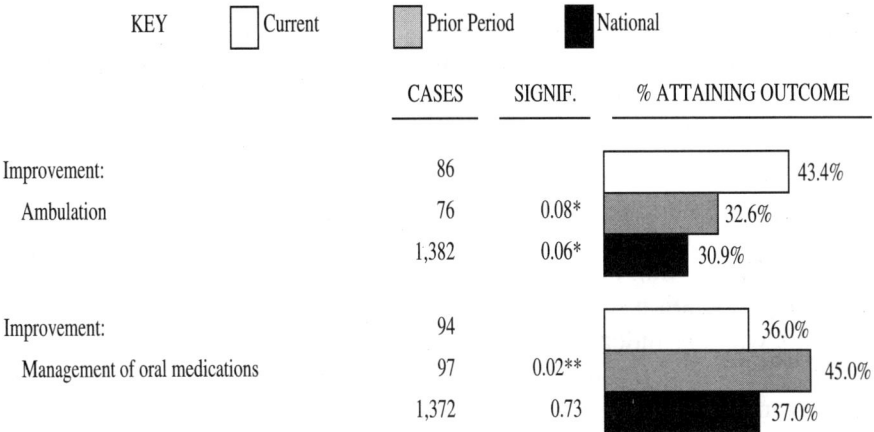

FIGURE 8.5. Excerpt from agency-level outcome report for orthopedic patients (hypothetical).

*The probability is 10% or less that this difference is due to chance, 90% or more that the difference is real.

**The probability is 5% or less that this difference is due to chance, 95% or more that the difference is real.

measures (from among several such measures) that pertain to orthopedic patients. Orthopedic conditions constitute one of the quality indicator groups or QUIGs. Improvement measures that correspond to end-result outcomes such as improvement in ambulation or improvement in management of oral medications as indicated in Figure 8.5, are constructed from health status scales at two points in time. In this case, the outcome measures correspond to change in ambulation status or ability to manage oral medications between start of care and discharge. The results indicate that 43.4% of orthopedic patients improved in ambulation during the current reporting period (most recent year) for the agency, compared with 32.6% of orthopedic patients for the agency's prior period (preceding year), and relative to 30.9% of patients from a national benchmark sample. Eighty-six orthopedic patients contributed to the outcome results in the current reporting period, and 76 contributed from the prior period; the national benchmark sample results are based on 1,382 orthopedic patients. The risk-adjusted comparison between the current and prior period outcomes resulted in a statistically significant difference between the two means (i.e., 43.4% vs. 32.6%, with $p = .08$). The risk-adjusted comparison with the national benchmark sample is significant at $p = .06$. An analogous statistical interpretation pertains for improvement in management of oral medications. The outcome reports routinely contain asterisked, double asterisked, or nonasterisked items, depending on whether the statistical significance occurs at the .10 level, .05 level, or not at all (i.e., $p > .10$).

Improvement outcome measures take on the value 1 if the patient improved according to the health status scale under consideration (in this case the ambulation scale and the management of oral medications scale). Patients who are independent or not disabled at the outset in terms of the health status under consideration are excluded from the computation of improvement measures because they cannot improve according to the scale under consideration. Analogously, although not shown in Figure 8.5, stabilization measures are used to reflect nonworsening in patient condition (i.e., either remaining the same or improving). For such measures, patients who are at the most disabled extreme of the health status scale are excluded because they cannot worsen. Therefore, floor and ceiling effects are addressed in this measure scheme through exclusion of patients at the floor or ceiling levels for the specific health status scales used to compute particular measures. A variety of different types of measures, several far more complex than the improvement or stabilization measures mentioned above, have been used for research purposes and tested for OBQI. However, from the viewpoint of clinical applicability and administrative simplicity, the improvement and stabilization measures presently appear to carry adequate information for purposes of changing care behaviors. Nonetheless, the OASIS data set permits continued experimentation with other types of outcome measures.

The purpose of the three-agency OBQI pilot in Colorado was to gain experience with OBQI in its initial stages. Funded by the Robert Wood Johnson Foundation, the goal was to implement primary data collection in three separate agencies using an initial data set that was later changed considerably, eventually becoming the OASIS after a series of iterations. The three agencies were provided selected types of outcomes reports and were allowed to conduct their second-stage screens in any manner they wished. The goal was to monitor how the three agencies might implement the OBQI approach rather than direct how they might do so. As a result of the demonstration (which continues), we have substantially modified the entire OBQI process in a variety of different ways. The data collection approach and methodologies are much more structured. Data items have become more specific, and outcome reporting entails more precise risk adjustment. A specific set of activities is now recommended for the second-stage screen. This approach is being further refined in the context of the national Medicare quality assurance demonstration mentioned above and is documented in two chapters in the OBQI manual mentioned earlier.

A number of practical issues have arisen in our initial OBQI work, resulting in a series of tips and practical pointers that can now be provided to agencies interested in implementing OBQI on their own (as well as those participating in the larger-scale demonstrations mentioned above). For example, we have learned that it is important not to permit providers of care to simply carry data items forward from SOC to follow-up points by providing information only on those items they feel have changed. This creates an incentive to minimize time spent collecting data at follow-up and inaccurately results in relatively few changes in patient status between admission and follow-up. When providers of care reassess health status at follow-up time points, considerably more changes are detected than if they are allowed to carry forward start-of-care health status items by default. The outcome reports for two pilot agencies were used to improve or change outcomes (demonstrated by subsequent outcome reports and reflected by substantial changes at the agency level that in turn had an effect on outcomes).

INTEGRATING OUTCOMES AND COST

As outcome measures and outcome measurement approaches continue to evolve, more widespread application of quality improvement using outcomes is likely. The aforementioned OBQI system for home care serves to illustrate this evolving trend. In view of the earlier conclusion that many of the key policy issues currently confronting us require a simultaneous evaluation of outcomes and costs of home care, the topic of cost monitoring or resource consumption reporting is germane to national policy deliberations on home care (Benjamin, 1992; Brody & Brody, 1989; Greenlick, 1988; Hughes, 1992; Miller, 1992; Rivlin & Wiener, 1988). An excerpt from an outcome report was provided in the preceding section. Figure 8.6 provides an illustrative excerpt from a resource consumption or cost report that can also be used at the agency level. Resource consumption reports can be generated to accompany outcome

182 Financing, Auspices, and Quality of Care

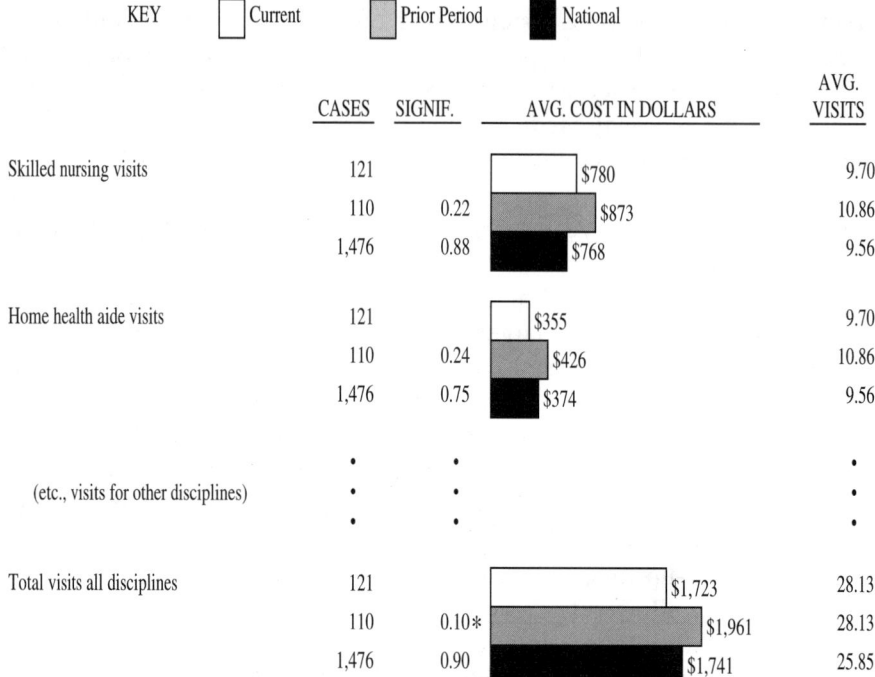

FIGURE 8.6. Excerpt from agency-level resource consumption (cost) report for orthopedic patients (hypothetical).

*The probability is 10% or less that this difference is due to chance, 90% or more that the difference is real.

**The probability is 5% or less that this difference is due to chance, 95% or more that the difference is real.

reports by collecting information on numbers of visits by discipline during the episode of care to which the outcome reports pertain (typically the interval between SOC and discharge). The excerpt from the resource consumption report in Figure 8.6 pertains to the same orthopedic patients in the current, prior, and national benchmark samples for which outcomes were computed to produce Figure 8.5. For the agency to which the reports pertain, a total of 121 orthopedic patients were involved in producing both Figures 8.5 and 6, although this is only apparent from examining Figure 8.6 where the number 121 appears in the column denoting current cases. For the outcome report in Figure 8.5, the exclusion criteria mentioned earlier were used (e.g., only 86 of the 121 orthopedic patients were impaired in ambulation, and therefore only 86 contributed to the computation of the outcome of improvement in ambulation). As is apparent from Figure 8.6, the average cost of skilled nursing visits per patient for the 121 orthopedic patients was $780, $873, and $768, respectively, corresponding to 9.70, 10.86, and 9.56—the average number of skilled nursing visits per patient for the current, prior, and national benchmark samples.* Analogous statistics are provided for home health aide visits. Although not shown in Figure 8.6, similar statistics can be produced for physical therapy visits, occupational therapy visits, speech/language pathology visits, medical social service visits, and so on. The last entry in Figure 8.6 presents total costs of $1,723, $1,961, and $1,741 for the current, prior, and national samples of orthopedic patients, respectively. Analogous statistics are presented for total visits.

CONCLUSION

We are at a unique point in the evolution of home care in the United States. A convergence of factors is occurring, both internal and external to the industry, that will guide and even reshape the provision of home care over the next decade (Riley, 1989; Weissert, Matthews, Cready, & Pawelak, 1988). Home care will move in the direction of per-episode prospective payment, increased penetration by managed care organizations, outcomes monitoring and management, and greater standardization of care processes. Over the next several years, progressively more comprehensive analyses of the cost and effectiveness of home care will be conducted (1) between and among different types of home care providers and (2) relative to other types of care (Hedrick & Inui, 1986; Kenney & Dubay, 1992; Kramer et al., 1997; Murdaugh, 1992). An essential ingredient for all such applications is a carefully and systematically derived set of data items that can be used to characterize the health status and care needs of patients at start of care and at regular time points thereafter, including discharge. Patient-level information on volume of services (visits) by discipline will also be essential for such analyses.

---

*It is possible to produce separate resource consumption reports for each outcome, using only those patients that contributed to the outcome computations. However, from a pragmatic perspective, a single resource consumption report based on all patients used for any outcome computations for the group under consideration (orthopedic patients in this case) is typically sufficient.

Therefore, as home care continues to grow and evolve, it should and will be analyzed more carefully in terms of its costs and benefits. As discussed at the beginning of this chapter, a vision or framework is needed that enables us to integrate cost and effectiveness issues in home care so that decisions and refinements in the provision of home care can be made at the levels of individual patients/clients, home care agencies, and the national home care delivery system, including integrating home care with other types of health care. In this regard, we first need a framework for concurrently evaluating cost and effectiveness of home care.

The outcome and resource consumption analyses and reports presented in the previous two sections constitute basic components of this framework. Such reports can provide information at both the agency level and the system level regarding outcomes and costs of home care. The framework should permit us to analyze cost and effectiveness for different types of patients/clients (i.e., according to different types of patient/client conditions or impairments, age groups, payer sources, etc.). Reporting mechanisms should allow for an evolution in both cost and outcome measures. Other types of quality measures in addition to outcome measures can and should be incorporated within the framework. Ultimately, we should reach a point where we can evaluate the cost of producing outcomes of various types, by patient condition. The types of outcome and resource consumption reports summarized earlier represent a step in this direction and could be reconfigured or reformatted as new measures emerge; as data items change or evolve; or as findings are presented at the subagency (e.g., branch, community, or departmental), multiagency, state, regional, or national levels.

Outcome reports can be expanded to include results on other quality measures. Figure 8.7 illustrates a report that incorporates various other types of quality measures (as well as outcomes). This report demonstrates how results can be displayed for end-result, utilization, and instrumental outcome measures. Although outcome measures are typically far more appropriate than process measures for CQI, this illustration also demonstrates how process measures can be incorporated into a holistic quality report. Even sentinel events can be incorporated into such a reporting scheme. For example, serious wound infections or malnutrition that result in hospitalization might be regarded as sentinel events to be reported in the manner shown in the lower portion of Figure 8.7. Thus, such a reporting format permits outcome monitoring using the more precise types of outcomes currently being employed in the ongoing OBQI

Agency: Utopia Home Health Services
Number of Patients in Current Period: 121
Number of Patients in Prior Period: 110

Prior period: 1/1/96–12/31/96
Report period: 1/1/97–12/31/97
Report date: 1/30/98

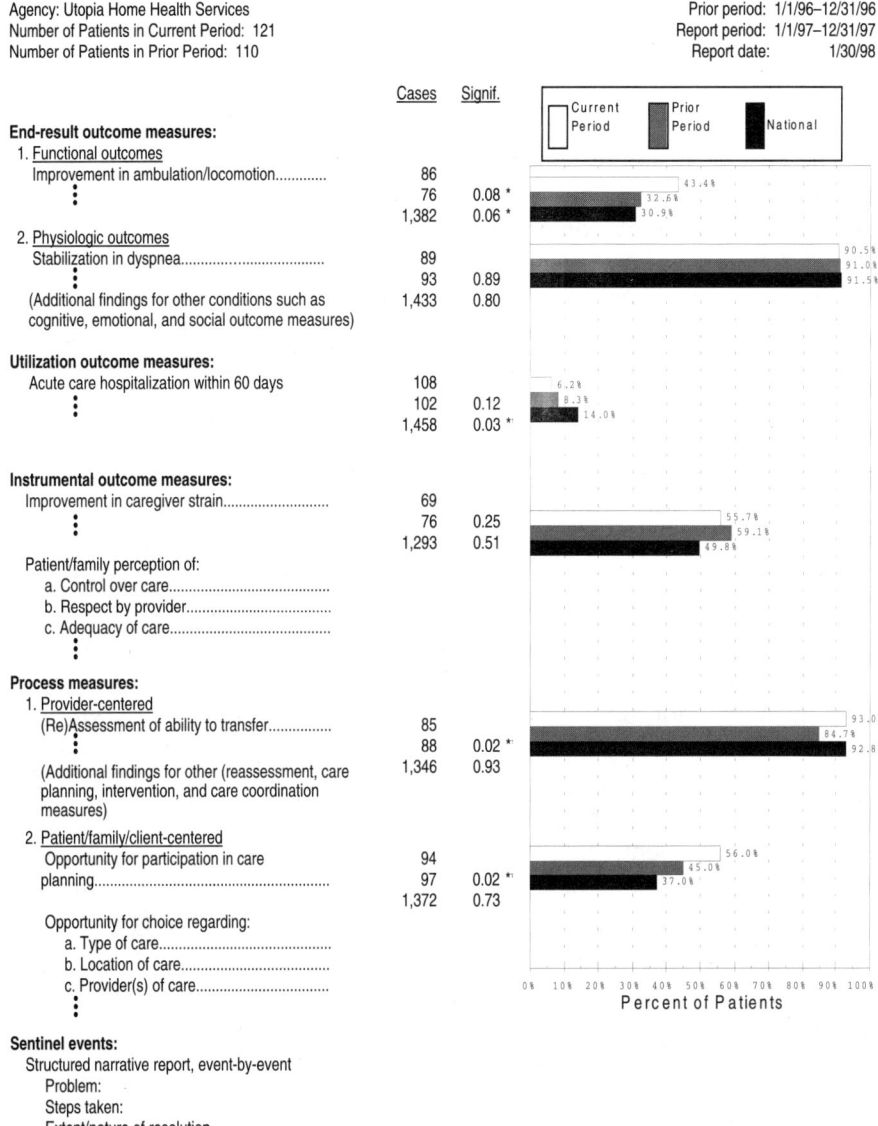

FIGURE 8.7. Risk-adjusted quality report for orthopedic patients/clients: quality and performance report on outcomes, processes of care, and sentinel events.

*The probability is 10% or less that this difference is due to chance, 90% or more that the difference is real.

**The probability is 5% or less that this difference is due to chance, 95% or more that the difference is real.

demonstration programs as well as different types of consumer-or client-centered quality measures that fall into the categories of either instrumental outcome or process measures. The more traditional sentinel-event reporting can also be incorporated into such a format.

The cost or resource consumption reports not only can be presented by patient type (e.g., condition or payer source), but can be further tailored to specific outcomes, so that the cost of producing specific outcomes for individual agencies or groups of agencies can be monitored. Furthermore, the manner in which resource consumption measures or costs are estimated can be progressively improved over time. For example, instead of estimating average cost per visit by discipline from agency-level (Medicare or other) cost reports, time per visit can be recorded and estimates of dollar-weighted time per visit computed for purposes of resource consumption reporting. These can be further refined by incorporating travel time, allocating indirect costs, and incorporating equipment/supply costs as appropriate. Thus, the aforementioned approach that concentrated on labor costs exclusively by imputing such costs from averages can and should be refined over time.

Above all, we should adhere to the principle that this cost-effectiveness framework must be useful and of practical value to individual home care agencies, not simply to payers or regulators. Without serving the needs of home care agencies in a practical sense, system-level reporting and monitoring activities will sink under their own weight. On the other hand, if a cost-effectiveness framework is of direct value for purposes of clinical management, quality improvement, case mix monitoring, cost monitoring, billing, and meeting regulatory and other fiscal requirements, the information and reporting system is likely to be diligently and accurately maintained by home care agency staff.

REFERENCES

Abt Associates Inc. (1995). *National home health agency prospective payment demonstration: Phase II: Procedures manual for home health agencies.* Cambridge, MA: Abt Associates Inc.

Benjamin, A. E. (1992). An overview of in-home health and supportive services for older persons. In M. G. Ory & A. P. Duncker (Eds.), *In-home care for older people: Health & supportive services* (pp. 9–52). Newbury Park, CA: Sage Publications.

Birnbaum, R. W. (1976). Health maintenance organizations: A guide to planning and development. New York: Spectrum Publications.
Brody, E. M., & Brody, S. J. (1989). The informal system of health care. In C. Eisdorfer, D. A. Kessler, & A. N. Spector (Eds.), *Caring for the elderly: Reshaping health policy* (pp. 259–277). Baltimore, MD: The Johns Hopkins University Press.
Christianson, J. (1980). The impact of HMOs: Evidence and research issues. *Journal of Health Politics, Policy and Law, 5,* 354–367.
Crisler, K S., Kramer, A. M., Jenkins, J., Bauman, M. K., Bostrom, S. G., & Shaughnessy, P. W. (1994). *Objective review criteria for abstracting data for clinical record review of home health care. Volume 3, Final report from: A study to develop outcome-based quality measures for home health services.* Denver: University of Colorado Health Sciences Center, Center for Health Services Research.
Enthoven, A. & Kronick, R. (1989a). A consumer-choice health plan for the 1990s: Universal health insurance in a system designed to promote quality and economy, Part 1. *New England Journal of Medicine, 320,* 29–37.
Enthoven, A., & Kronick, R. (1989b). A consumer-choice health plan for the 1990s: Universal health insurance in a system designed to promote quality and economy, Part 2. *New England Journal of Medicine, 320,* 94–101.
Fries, B. E., Schneider, D. P., Foley, W. J., Gavazzi, M., Burke, R., & Cornelius, E. (1994). Refining a case-mix measure for nursing homes: Resource Utilization Groups (RUG-III). *Medical Care, 32,* 668–685.
Granger, C. V., & Clark, G. S. (1994). Functional status and outcomes of stroke rehabilitation. *Topics in Geriatric Rehabilitation, 9* (3), 72–84.
Granger, C. V. & Hamilton, B. B. (1990). Measurement of stroke rehabilitation outcome in the 1980s. [Review] *Stroke, 21* (9 Suppl.), 1146–1147.
Granger, C. V., Hamilton, B. B., Linacre, J. M., Heinemann, A. W., & Wright, B. D. (1993). Performance profiles of the functional independence measure. *American Journal of Physical Medicine & Rehabilitation, 72* (2), 84–89.
Granger, C., Kelley-Hayes, M., Johnston M., Deutsch, A., Braun, S., & Fiedler, R. (1996). Quality and outcome measures in medical rehabilitation. In R. Braddom (Ed.), *Physical medicine and rehabilitation* (pp. 239–253). Philadelphia: W. B. Saunders.
Granger, C. V., Ottenbacher, K. J., & Fiedler, R. C. (1995). The Uniform Data System for medical rehabilitation: Report of first admissions for 1993. *American Journal of Physical Medicine & Rehabilitation, 74* (1), 62–66.
Greenlick, M. (1988). The S/HMO demonstration: Policy implications for long-term care in HMOs. *Pride Institute Journal of Long Term Home Health Care, 7* (3), 15–24.
Greenspun, B. (1994). Putting outcome data to use. Protocol for stroke rehabilitation based on outcome data. *Advance/Rehabilitation, 3* (5), 47–49.

Hawes, C., Morris, J. N., Phillips, C. D., Mor, V., Fries, B. E., & Nonemaker, S. (1995). Reliability estimates for the Minimum Data Set for nursing home resident assessment and care screening (MDS). *Gerontologist, 35,* 172–78.

Hedrick, S. C., & Inui, T. S. (1986). The effectiveness and cost of home care: An information synthesis. *Health Services Research, 20,* 851–880.

Hughes, S. L. (1992). Home care: Where we are and where we need to go. In M. G. Ory & A. P. Duncker (Eds.), *In-home care for older people: Health and supportive services* (pp. 53–74). Newbury Park, CA: Sage Publications.

Kenney, G. M., & Dubay, L. C. (1992). Explaining area variation in the use of Medicare home health services. *Medical Care, 30* (1), 43–57.

Kramer, A. M., Shaughnessy, P. W., Bauman, M. K., & Crisler, K S. (1990). Assessing and assuring the quality of home health care: A conceptual framework. *Milbank Quarterly, 68,* 413–443.

Kramer, A. M., Steiner, J. F., Schlenker, R. E., Eilertsen, T. B., Hrincevich, C. A., Tropea, D. A., Ahmad, L. A., & Eckhoff, D. G. (1997). Outcomes and costs after hip fracture and stroke: A comparison of rehabilitation settings. *Journal of the American Medical Association, 277*(5), 396–404.

Lohr, K. N., & Schroeder, S. A. (1990). A strategy for quality assurance in Medicare. *New England Journal of Medicine, 322,* 707–712.

Miller, N. A. (1992). Medicaid 2176 home and community-based care waivers: The first ten years. *Health Affairs, 11*(4), 162–171.

Morris, J. N., Hawes, C., Fries, B. E., Phillips, C. D., Mor, V., Katz, S., Murphy, K., Drugovich, M. L., & Friedlob, A. S. (1990). Designing the national resident assessment instrument for nursing homes. *Gerontologist, 30,* 293–307.

Morrison, E. M., & Luft, H. S. (1990). Health maintenance organization environments in the 1980s and beyond. *Health Care Financing Review, 12*(1), 81–90.

Murdaugh, C. (1992). Quality of life, functional status, patient satisfaction. *Patient outcomes research: Examining the effectiveness of nursing practice,* (NIH-93-3411). Bethesda, MD: U.S. Public Health Service.

National Association for Home Care. (1995). Medicare's OASIS: Standardized outcome and assessment information set for home health care. *NAHC Report* (Suppl. 625).

Powell, M. C., Shaughnessy, P. W., Schlenker, R. E., Crisler, K. S., Hittle, D. F., Kramer, A. M., Beale, S. K., Bostrom, S. G., Beaudry, J. M., DeVore, P. A., Spencer, M. J., Chandramouli, V., Grant, W. V., Arnold, A. G., Bauman, M. K., & Jenkins, J. (1994). Technical appendices to the report on measuring outcomes of home health care (Vol. 2). A study to develop outcome-based quality measures for home health services. Denver: Univer-

sity of Colorado Health Sciences Center, Center for Health Services Research.
Riley, P. A. (1989). *Quality assurance in home care.* Washington, DC: American Association of Retired Persons.
Rivlin, A. M., & Wiener, J. M., with Hanley, R. J., & Spence, D. A. (1988). *Caring for the disabled elderly: Who will pay?* Washington DC: The Brookings Institution.
Schlenker, R. E. (1996). *Home health payment legislation: Review and recommendations.* Washington, DC: American Association for Retired Persons, Division of Legislation and Public Policy, Public Policy Institute.
Schlenker, R. E., Shaughnessy, P. W., & Hittle, D. F. (1995). Patient-level cost of home health care under capitated and fee-for-service payment. *Inquiry, 32*(3), 252–270.
Shaughnessy, P. W. (1991). *Shaping policy for long-term care: Learning from the effectiveness of hospital swing beds.* Ann Arbor: Health Administration Press.
Shaughnessy, P. W., & Crisler, K. S., with Arnold, A., Beaudry, J., Powell, M., DeVore, P., Hittle, D., Schlenker, R., Kramer, A., Bostrom, S., & Campbell, B. (1995). *Outcome-based quality improvement: A manual for home care agencies on how to use outcomes.* Washington, DC: National Association for Home Care.
Shaughnessy, P. W., Crisler, K. S., & Kramer, A. M. (1989). Quality of care indicators in home care: Preliminary indicators and directions for future research (Study Paper No. 2). Denver: University of Colorado Health Sciences Center, Center for Health Services Research.
Shaughnessy, P. W., Crisler, K. S., Schlenker, R. E., & Arnold, A. G. (1995). Outcome-based quality improvement in home care. *Caring, 14*(2), 44–49.
Shaughnessy, P. W., Crisler, K. S., Schlenker, R. E., Arnold, A. G., Kramer, A. M., Powell, M. C., & Hittle, D. F. (1994). Measuring and assuring the quality of home care. *Health Care Financing Review, 16*(1), 35–68.
Shaughnessy, P. W., Schlenker, R. E., Crisler, K. N., Arnold, A. G., Powell, M. C., & Beaudry, J. M. (1996). Home health care: Moving forward with continuous quality improvement, *Journal of Aging and Social Policy, 7* (3/4), 149–167, and in M. E. Cowart, & J. Quadagno (Eds.), *From nursing homes to home care* (pp. 149–167). Binghamton, NY: Haworth Press.
Shaughnessy, P. W., Schlenker, R. E., Crisler, K. S., Powell, M. C., Hittle, D. F., Kramer, A. M., Spencer, M. J., Beale, S. K., Bostrom, S. G., Beaudry, J. M., DeVore, P. A., Chandramouli, V., Grant, W. V., Arnold, A. G., Bauman, M. K., & Jenkins, J. (1994). *Measuring outcomes of home health care* (Vol. 1). Denver: Center for Health Policy Research.
Shaughnessy, P. W., Schlenker, R. E., & Hittle, D. F. (1995). Case mix of home health patients under capitated and fee-for-service payment. *Health Services Research, 30*(1), 79–113.

Shaughnessy, P. W., Schlenker, R. E., Hittle, D. F., with Kramer, A. M., Crisler, K. S., Spencer, M. J., DeVore, P. A., Grant, W. V., Beaudry, J. M., & Chandramouli, V. (1994). *Study of home health care quality and cost under capitated and fee-for-service payment systems: Technical report* (Vol. 2). Denver: Center for Health Policy Research.

State University of New York at Buffalo. (1993). *Guide to the Uniform Data Set for Medical Rehabilitation (Adult FIMsm) version 4.0*. Buffalo: Author.

State University of New York at Buffalo. (1995). *Getting started with the Uniform Data System for Medical Rehabilitation (Adult FIMsm)*. Buffalo: Author.

Weissert, W. G., Matthews Cready, C., & Pawelak, J. E. (1988). Past and future of home-and community-based long-term care. *Milbank Quarterly, 66,* 309–388.

CHAPTER 9

Testing Home Care as a Managed Care Intervention

Susan L. Hughes
Frances M. Weaver

Home health care currently is receiving unprecedented public scrutiny, largely as a result of double-digit increases that occurred annually in Medicare home health care expenditures between 1991 and 1997 (see chapter 1). As a result of these increases, Medicare home health care has became the fastest growing component of personal health care expenditures (Komisar & Feder, 1998). In response, the Balanced Budget Act of 1997 attempted to rein in expenditures through fairly draconian measures. Beginning in 1998 average reimbursements to home care programs were reduced from actual costs up to a cap based on 112% of the national average cost per visit, to 105% of the national median per-visit cost, and annual per patient spending was capped at specific amounts, depending on a patient's age and location (U.S. General Accounting Office, 1998). This interim payment system, which is scheduled to be replaced by prospective payment in the near future, penalizes agencies that have been more frugal by basing current caps on prior billings. Thus, those agencies that provided fewer visits and billed less in the past report are being hardest hit.

The dramatic increase in home health expenditures from 1991 to 1997 reflected several factors, including the expansion of Medicare home care regulations in the early 1980s to allow proprietary providers in states without licensure to participate in the program; the elimination of the eligibility requirement of a 3-day prior hospitalization; the implementation of prospective payment to hospitals, which encouraged the discharge of patients "quicker and sicker"; and the loosening of regulations concerning limits on visits, resulting from a class action law suit in 1989 (Bishop & Skwara, 1993). As a result of these changes, the composition of Medicare home care providers changed substantially, with major growth occurring in the number of hospital-based and proprietary programs (Hughes, 1991). Simultaneously, the home care industry has been coping with significant increases in the acuity level of patients served, the provision of increasingly complex technological care (see chapter 3), and the inroads of managed care.

Although the Medicare home health care benefit was originally intended to reduce use of hospital days, a national study of geographic variation in use of the benefit, by Welch, Wennberg, and Welch (1996), found that only 57% of home care users had been hospitalized during the 6–month period prior to receiving home care and found no relationship between level of home care use and reduction of hospital days. According to the authors, these findings again raise important questions about the current targeting of the Medicare home health care benefit to persons at risk of a high cost outcome.

What the Welch and colleagues article did not do, however, was address the issue of how the provision of care to high risk patients, once identified, should be *managed.* Indeed, very little literature has appeared on this issue despite the fact that high-risk patients frequently have complex, medically unstable conditions that pose significant challenges for care coordination and continuity. Within this policy context, *tests of innovative home care management models* are sorely needed. This chapter attempts to meet that need by describing some recent demonstrations/ studies of home care innovations provided by hospital-based home care management teams in the Chicago metropolitan area. Unlike the customary provision of home care, these programs involve the specific targeting of high-risk patients with ongoing primary care management provided directly by the home care team, including direct hands on involvement of the home care physician, or the explicit use of condition-specific home care protocols that were developed jointly by home care staff and relevant physician specialists

The chapter begins by summarizing what is currently known about home care cost effectiveness. Then it describes three randomized studies (one completed and two ongoing) testing the capacity of the above-referenced home care management models. The pivotal role of the physician as an active member of the home care team in all three studies is discussed, and, finally, the implications of these studies for home care research and policy are considered.

HOME CARE COST EFFECTIVENESS

Despite general consensus that home care is here to stay, controversy persists in the literature regarding its cost effectiveness (Kemper, Applebaum, & Harrigan, 1988). Part of this controversy stems from the fact that home care was subjected to summative outcome studies very early, while still a new service modality. This concentration on outcomes reflected policymakers' concerns regarding home care cost effectiveness. Given the rapid growth in home care programs, clients, and expenditures, policymakers wanted to know the impact of home care on total health care costs. In turn, providers somewhat rashly promised cost savings that could be achieved by substituting home care for costly institutional care. As a result of premature but understandably zealous pursuit of evidence showing an impact on cost, policymakers, providers, and evaluators rushed to conduct summative evaluations, before articulating theories about how these new services could be expected to work and why. Consequently, we have experienced 25 to 30 years of summative evaluations of a wide array of community-based interventions (some home care and some not) that have produced very contradictory findings concerning effectiveness (Hedrick & Inui, 1986; Hughes, 1985; Kemper et al., 1988; Weissert, Cready & Pawelak, 1988).

In our view, the conflicting research findings to date largely reflect the lack of a coherent theoretical approach to the study of home care. Take, for example, the National Long Term Care Demonstration (also known as the Channeling Demonstration). This multisite demonstration was intended to provide an unequivocal answer to the "substitution" question. In other words, this study was intended to determine whether case-managed community care saved money by substituting home/community-based long-term care for more expensive hospital or nursing home care (Kemper et al., 1988).

Unfortunately, people who designed the evaluation did not spend enough time thinking through in advance how and why Channeling would have an impact on hospital and nursing home use. If they had developed a logic model, spelling out how the intervention would work before implementing the evaluation, they might have realized something very important—nurses and social work case management teams do not make decisions to hospitalize or institutionalize people. Rather, these decisions are made by patients, patients' families, and physicians. Thus, a community-based intervention that consists of a nurse/social work team that does not include active physician participation is not likely to affect hospital or nursing home use. In fact, that is what the evaluation found. Specifically, although case management improved clients' satisfaction with care, reduced clients' unmet service needs, and made clients more confident that their needs would be met, it did not reduce hospital or nursing home admissions in the treatment group vis-à-vis the control group. A competing interpretation of these findings is that the evaluation design and the intervention suffered from theory failure (e.g., inadequate specification of the means through which the new program would achieve its desired outcomes).

Other earlier evaluations of community-based care also suffered from conceptual flaws. For example, the Community Care Organization in Wisconsin attempted to test the impact of case-managed home-and community-based care on people who were at high risk of nursing home admission (Applebaum, Seidl, & Austin, 1980). Because the state of Wisconsin was mainly interested in reducing Medicaid nursing home expenditures, the demonstration was limited to clients in the community who were already Medicaid-eligible. As a result, the demonstration targeted a young-old population that bears little resemblance to the typical nursing home population. The evaluators did not realize that their real at-risk population was elderly and disabled people with poor social supports living in the community who were not receiving Medicaid but who would become Medicaid eligible after they spent down their resources during their first few months of nursing home use. Thus, in addition to having a defensible theory about how and why the program will work, it is also necessary to know what population should be targeted to receive the intervention and why (Hughes, 1985).

Although much of the home care effectiveness literature exhorts providers to target services to high-risk populations, this charge can be realized only if we take the time to ask, At high risk of what? and What resources does the program have that can be reasonably expected to affect that outcome? For example, home care currently encompasses at least four different major models—high tech, Medicare skilled, low-tech homemaker/chore /personal care services, and hospice (Hughes, 1991). Although it may be reasonable to expect that high-tech, Medicare skilled home care, and hospice care could reduce hospital admissions and/or days, it is likely that low-tech home care would have more of an affect on reducing nursing home admissions and/or days.

Below, we illustrate the importance of a conceptual modeling approach to home care evaluations with examples of three studies that address the relationship between patient targeting, services provided, and outcomes that can be posited as being likely given patient targeting and program service characteristics.

HOME CARE IN THE DEPARTMENT OF VETERANS AFFAIRS

The Department of Veterans Affairs (DVA) health care system encompasses 172 health care facilities nationally. Approximately 73 of the larger hospitals in the system currently have contracts to provide Home Based Primary Care (HBPC), which previously was titled Hospital Based Home Care (HBHC). HBPC differs from the Medicare home health care benefit in that it is funded prospectively as part of each participating hospital's budget. In 1983 staff at the Edward F. Hines, Jr. VA Hospital HBHC program in Hines, Illinois, wanted to learn whether the program was saving the DVA money by targeting and serving two high-risk patient groups. One group was severely disabled persons with two or more impairments in activities of daily living (ADLs) at the time of hospital discharge. The other was persons who were terminally ill (those with a prognosis of less than 6 months survival time). The Hines model was unique at that time within the DVA with respect to its use of these patient targeting criteria *and* its ability to provide continuous team-managed home care, including physician care, within and outside the acute care setting. The staff believed that they were providing effective care for these patients and were saving the DVA money. We submitted a proposal to conduct a randomized trial to test this assumption and were funded to do so in the early 1980s.

The Hines HBHC study examined cost effectiveness by prospectively screening all acute admissions to the 1,100–bed Hines facility over a 3-year period to identify and randomize 233 severely disabled veteran and informal caregiver pairs and 171 terminally ill veteran and informal caregiver pairs to HBHC or to customary care. Findings from this study included significant increases in patient and caregiver satisfaction with HBHC care that were accompanied by net cost savings of 10% in the severely disabled group and 18% in the terminally ill group, yielding a net cost savings of 13% (Cummings et al., 1990; Hughes et al., 1990, 1992). Although this net cost savings was not statistically significant, it is the largest cost savings reported to date in the home care literature. Importantly, the savings were largely attributable to reductions in hospital readmission days and to use of lower intensity hospital beds within a hospital stay. As a result, cost of readmission hospital care was 24% lower in the severely disabled intervention group and 39.5% lower in the terminally ill intervention group, yielding a significant hospital readmission cost savings of 29% ($p = .03$) for the two groups combined.

Interestingly, different dynamics were seen by study subgroup with respect to how this savings in hospital readmission costs was achieved. Although no difference was seen in rate of hospital readmission by group among terminally ill patients, the terminally ill treatment group used significantly fewer readmission days. Specifically, when terminally ill treatment group patients were readmitted to the hospital, they tended to be very close to death, frequently within 24 to 48 hours. These patients were already known to the HBHC physician, who often continued to serve as their attending physician during hospital readmissions. The HBHC physician also directed the hospital inpatient intermediate care step-down unit. Thus, the HBHC physician could manage the care of these patients in the community, continue to manage their care in the hospital during their last days of life, and could place these patients in lower cost step-down beds without compromising the quality of their medical care. Terminally ill control patients, in contrast, tended to be admitted 1 to 2 weeks before dying in the hospital and remained in acute care beds for the duration of the admission.

Among the severely disabled participants, again, no group difference was observed in rate of hospital readmission, but treatment patients tended to be rehospitalized almost exclusively in the VA, whereas at least some control group patients used private sector hospitals that were more expensive. Again, severely disabled treatment group patients who were rehospitalized in the VA were moved by the HBHC physician to a step-down unit as soon as possible, whereas control group patients who were hospitalized either in private sector hospitals or at Hines tended to stay in an acute bed for the duration of their stay.

Thus, the HBHC model at Hines primarily succeeded in reducing costs because the physician, working with the home care team, was able to manage the patient's care and strategic resources like the hospital step-down unit continuously in and outside of the hospital. Because of these features, we called the Hines model Team Managed/Hospital Based Home Care (TM/HBHC). Although the findings from this single-site study suggested that this model had the potential to reduce costs of care while simultaneously increasing patient and caregiver satisfaction, a trial with substantially more patients and additional sites was necessary to definitively test the effect of the model on costs and to assess the model's generalizability in the DVA. These issues are currently being addressed in a DVA cooperative study of TM/HBHC.

VA COOPERATIVE STUDY OF TM/HBHC

The cooperative TM/HBHC study began in October 1994 and involves replicating and testing the TM/HBHC model at 16 DVA hospitals across the country with a sample of 1,800 patients (Cummings, Hughes, & Weaver, 1992). The study's primary objective is to determine whether treatment group patients experience significantly lower total health care costs, primarily as a function of reduced hospital readmission costs. Secondary outcomes include patient functional status, patient and informal caregiver health-related quality of life (Ware & Sherbourne, 1992), patient and caregiver satisfaction with care, and caregiver burden (Montgomery, Gonyea, & Hooyman, 1985). Patients were recruited to the study during an acute hospital admission, stratified by age and by diagnostic group, and randomized to either TM/HBHC or to customary care, which can include any other services exclusive of HBHC in the DVA and any services in the community to which they are entitled. Patients who were assigned to the control group were encouraged by the study staff to speak with their VA physician or discharge planner about alternative plans for after care. All study participants were assessed at baseline, 1

Table 9.1 Components of TM/HBHC Intervention

1. Interdisciplinary team includes physician with admitting privileges.
2. Targets high hospital users.
3. Designated care manager.
*4. Complete patient assessments and comprehensive care plans.
5. Twenty-four–hour telephone coverage for night/weekend emergencies.
6. Prior authorization by HBHC physician or designate for nonemergency hospital admissions/clinic use; HBHC staff consult with inpatient team, facilitate prompt transfer of patients to less intensive beds, and early discharge planning.
*7. Weekly team meeting and 90–day minimum patient clinical and utilization review, including consideration of suitability for discharge.

*Routine elements of care that are included in the VA HBHC Guidelines.

month, 6 months and 12 months. Health services use and cost data are being obtained from automated DVA and Health Care Financing Administration (HCFA) claims databases whenever possible and supplemented when necessary with patient utilization information recorded in patient diaries and subsequently confirmed in writing or by telephone by research staff with providers.

Before the study began, the study protocol delineated the components of the TM/HBHC model. Table 9.1 displays the seven components of the model and indicates that two were already included in the VA HBHC Program guidelines. These components are starred and consist of fairly traditional requirements like presence of an interdisciplinary team, weekly team meetings, and minimum 90–day patient reviews. Importantly, HBHC differs from the Medicare model in stipulating that the interdisciplinary team include a physician. We strengthened that component further by stipulating that the physician have hospital admitting privileges. In addition, we added four new requirements that were intended to capture the way the HBHC program was managed at Hines.

First, we stipulated that the program must target persons at *high risk of hospital use* (e.g., the severely disabled and the terminally ill). When this cooperative study began, HBHC programs were funded prospectively as part of each hospital director's overall budget and considerable discretion was left to the facility with respect to targeting the service. Second, we specified that the program must *designate a care manager for each patient*. Third, we specified that the program *must provide 24–*

hour telephone coverage for night or weekend emergencies. Finally, we also specified that the *HBHC physician/physician designate authorize all nonemergency rehospitalizations* for active TM/HBHC patients, that the TM/HBHC team track all hospital readmissions, institute communication and discharge planning, and use step-down units whenever possible. At the time that these components were identified (early 1990s) the DVA offered very little ongoing primary care management to patients. Thus, these home care guidelines were somewhat revolutionary in nature.

At present, we are close to the end of the cooperative study. To date, 1,967 patients have been enrolled in the study at 16 DVA hospitals across the United States. We have learned a number of lessons as a result of implementing the study and have had to modify the study protocol several times since the study began.

Although the study inclusion criteria originally were limited to severely disabled and terminally ill patients, we have learned that hospice care is much more readily available now to veterans both within the DVA and in the community than it was in the 1980s, when we conducted the first Hines study. Therefore, participating study sites have had a more difficult time enrolling the same proportion of terminally ill patients that was enrolled in the earlier study. Whereas the proportion of terminally ill patients in the earlier study was 30%, it is 20% in the current cooperative study. Because cost savings in the earlier study were especially pronounced in the terminally ill subgroup, we have sought to replace terminally ill patients by expanding the inclusion criteria to include other high risk groups—namely, patients with congestive heart failure (CHF) or chronic obstructive pulmonary disease (COPD) who are homebound. Currently, the latter two groups constitute another 5% of study enrollees.

Current DVA guidelines for cooperative studies in health services mandate that study investigators be blinded to study outcomes while data collection is ongoing in the field. Therefore, we have only recently become privy to outcomes broken down by study group. Preliminary findings indicate that the study sample is 75% disabled, 20% terminally ill, and 5% CHF or COPD. The majority (80%) of patients is over age 65, with a mean age of 72. The great majority (96%) of participants is male, 65% are white, and one third of participants has annual incomes less than $10,000. DVA HBHC regulations stipulate that all participants have some type of informal caregiver involved in their care. The majority of participants in our study (82%) reside with a caregiver who, in the majority of instances, is a spouse (57%) or child (17%). Importantly, with respect to retrospective risk, 88% of participants had experienced a prior hospitalization during the six months prior to study entry, and no significant differences have been detected between the study treatment and control groups at baseline. Because we are still merging VA and HCFA claims data for the last two years of the study, no cost estimates are available at this time.

Private Sector Study

Because the generalizability of the DVA TM/HBHC managed home care model to the private health care sector is currently unknown, we have adapted it for use and testing in the private sector. We believe that the TM/HBHC model succeeded in the DVA because it encourages physician involvement in managing patient care. When we conducted the first HBHC study in the 1980s, VA physicians had no financial incentive to retain patients in their practices because they are salaried. Therefore, it was possible for the primary care management of VA HBHC patients to be transferred from the admitting physician to the HBHC physician for ongoing care management inside and outside of the hospital. While the current cooperative study was being conducted, the VA moved to more of a capitated approach to physician reimbursement; however, anecdotal evidence from TM/HBHC program managers indicates that physicians generally do not object to transferring primary care to the TM/HBHC physician, in large part, because these patients are inherently difficult to manage. Generally, the HBHC physician does not make frequent home visits to active patients but is available to review patients with the home care team, to visit patients at home as necessary, and to facilitate planned versus emergency hospital readmissions to the maximum extent possible.

Incentives for physician involvement in Medicare home health care are quite different. Under the fee-for-service Medicare home health care regulations, patient referrals must emanate from a physician. Although most Medicare-certified programs either have access to a physician consultant or have a medical director, this individual usually performs in a consulting capacity because the referring physician usually prefers to retain primary care management. In reality, however, the referring physician's actual role in home care treatment can be quite minimal. Frequently, physicians discharge patients to a home care provider at the discharge planner's request. After home care begins, the burden of provider/physician communication about the patient's condition is assumed by the home care provider. Medicare requires home health care providers to obtain physician recertification of the patient's continued need for care 60 days following the start of care. However, little is known about the pattern and quality of communication that takes place between home care providers and the large number of physicians who can be responsible for patients receiving home care on any given day. In fact, until 1993, Medicare actually discouraged physician involvement in home care by setting payment for physician home visits at a lower rate than that of home health aides (Rust, 1992). The reimbursement rate has since been raised to $81 if the home care management requires more than 30 minutes of a physician's time. However, the documentation that is required for reimbursement has deterred many physicians from billing for this service.

In response to this problem, the American Medical Association has developed and disseminated generic physician home care practice guidelines. Also, increasing numbers of home care providers have hired medical directors to interface with referring physicians when necessary and to provide medical guidance for nursing staff. Although both of these developments are probably helpful, they may not be sufficient to ensure optimal patient care outcomes, given the increasing complexity and severity of medical conditions treated in the home.

In order to develop and test a TM/HBHC model for use in the private sector, we held extensive discussions with the administrators and physicians of Northwestern Memorial Home Health Care, Inc. (NMHHC), the hospital-linked subsidiary that provides home health care services for patients discharged from Northwestern Memorial Hospital. We discussed the features of the TM/HBHC model with NMHHC staff and examined NMHHC's organizational structure, physician referral patterns, and patient utilization data. The utilization data indicated that NMHHC provided care to substantial numbers of patients with total joint replacements (TJR) of the hip (THR) or knee (TKR) and to patients with congestive heart failure (CHF). A test of the TM/HBHC model with these particular patient groups is particularly interesting because our theory suggests that these two groups, both of whom are high-volume users of health care, would experience very different home care outcomes.

TJR patients undergo an elective hospitalization for a surgical procedure that requires substantial amounts of postdischarge physical therapy. Although both joint replacement procedures are widely acknowledged to be successful, at present we do not know what effect postdischarge care has on functional status and cost outcomes. When our study began, 36% of THR patients and 39% of TKR patients hospitalized at Northwestern Memorial Hospital received short-term rehabilitation hospital care for approximately 7 days following discharge at a cost of approximately $1,000 per day. If a rehab bed was not available, patients were retained in the hospital for an additional 1 to 2 days of acute care. The two surgeons who perform the majority of the TJR procedures have worked with NMHHC to develop a protocol for the aftercare of TJR patients in the home. Because of the high cost of inpatient rehabilitation hospital stays (the aggregate in fiscal year 1992 was estimated, at a minimum, to be $775,000), the surgeons wanted to learn whether a TJR home care protocol that provided more intensive therapy in the first weeks after hospital discharge could substitute for and/or reduce rehabilitation hospital days (thereby reducing costs) and simultaneously produce the same or better functional status outcomes.

In contrast to THR, CHF is a potentially life-threatening condition that accounts for more hospital discharges than any other diagnosis-related group (Kantrowitz, 1988). Most patients who are hospitalized for treatment of CHF have a New York Heart Association Functional Class score of 3 or 4 (Criteria Committee of the New York Heart Association, 1964). Patients with class 3 cardiac disease experience marked limitation of physical activity. Although these patients are comfortable at rest, less than ordinary activity causes fatigue, palpitation, dyspnea, or anginal pain. Class 4 patients cannot carry on any physical activity without discomfort, and symptoms may even be present at rest.

A 1985 study of 6-month hospital readmission rates among patients 65 years of age and older found that patients with a primary diagnosis of CHF were at higher risk of hospital readmission than patients with cerebrovascular disease or hip fracture (Gooding & Jette, 1985). Patients with CHF who were admitted for a short stay and discharged directly home and those with atrial and ventricular arrhythmias and uncorrected valve defects were at particular risk. According to the authors, "[M]ore aggressive home care after discharge, improved coordination efforts with primary care provider, frequent monitoring, or increased use of step-down facilities such as rehabilitation hospitals might substantially reduce readmission for related causes for this cohort" (p. 600).

As this brief review indicates, both persons with TJR surgery and persons hospitalized with a primary diagnosis of CHF appear to be appropriate target populations for a skilled home care intervention. Both patient populations are eligible for Medicare-reimbursed home health care. It seems reasonable that a skilled, team-managed hospital-linked home care (TM/HLHC) model that maximizes physician input into the development of condition-specific protocols would be most successful for these patient groups. Consistent with our theory, different utilization outcomes are likely for the two groups. Specifically, we hypothesized that the provision of TM/HLHC to patients following TJR would reduce short-term rehabilitation hospital admissions. In contrast, TM/HLHC is expected to reduce acute hospital readmission days for the CHF group. These savings were hypothesized to be accompanied by similar or improved patient functional status outcomes, using both generic and condition-specific measures.

We received NIH funding to begin a randomized study of TM/HLHC for CHF and TJR patients in 1994. The first year of the study was devoted to developing the condition-specific home care protocols with teams of physicians and home care staff and pilot tests of patient enrollment systems. Currently, both arms of the study are up and running. Approximately 137 CHF patients and 135 TJR patients have been enrolled. It has been incredibly challenging conducting this type of study in the current chaotic health care environment. For example, we discovered in year 1 of the study that at least 200 different physicians currently admit CHF patients to our large teaching hospital. This meant that we had to provide numerous presentations regarding the study protocol to several different attending and house staff physician groups in addition to holding meetings with discharge planners and other hospital staff who needed to be involved in implementing the study protocol.

We have also encountered Medicare reimbursement and regulatory obstacles with respect to implementing the home care protocols. For example, CHF patients frequently are admitted to the hospital from the emergency room. Because their electrolytes become unbalanced at home, they begin to accumulate fluid, have difficulty breathing, and are admitted to the hospital from the emergency room in crisis. If patients were routinely discharged home with supplies of lasix or some other diuretic that could be administered intravenously on an as-needed basis, by the home care nurse after consultation with the physician and/or based on preset parameters regarding same, this type of emergency admission could be prevented. However, despite their low cost (approximately $10 for a 1-month supply), at present Medicare will not reimburse for diuretics to be stored in the home. Moreover, because Medicare does not reimburse for high-tech home care, most agencies have set up separate corporate entities to handle their Medicare and high-tech enterprises. Thus, it is difficult to have the same home care nurse provide continuous care to the CHF patient despite the fact that continuity of care is critically important from a clinical perspective for these high-risk patients.

CONCLUSION

As this chapter demonstrates, hospital-based and/or -linked home care programs come in all shapes and sizes and vary considerably in terms of patient targeting and scope, intensity, and complexity of services provided. Thus, the specific characteristics of a home care intervention must be clearly understood before any attempt is made to evaluate or test it.

From a policy perspective, we as a society face many challenges in our attempts to design a home care benefit that can respond flexibly to the realities of today's rapidly changing health care environment. We do not have a clear consensus about appropriate targeting criteria for the skilled home care benefit, and we have learned that fee-for-service reimbursement encourages over utilization. However, early returns from studies of home care provided by managed care plans for Medicare beneficiaries are not encouraging. Work by Shaughnessy, Schlenker, and Hittle (1994), for example, indicates that managed care plans reduce home care utilization and costs, but at the expense of poorer patient functional status outcomes. Prospective payment for home care, soon to be implemented by Medicare, holds some hope of constraining the current rate of increase in home care expenditures. Yet we believe it will be important to design flexible regulations that facilitate the continuous involvement and management of clinical care by physicians as active members of an interdisciplinary home care team if we are to maximize patient outcomes. In other words, it is not the home care benefit, but the way the benefit is managed that is key. Early returns based on the work by Shaughnessy and colleagues indicate that Medicare managed care plans are contracting out home care to existing home care providers and being even more parsimonious than Medicare with respect to utilization review of the benefit. These findings indicate that managed care plans have yet to discover the unique potential that home care might provide with respect to managing the care of high-risk patients cost effectively.

Because managed care plans can provide care more flexibly than Medicare agencies can, they are in an enviable position regarding opportunities to experiment with innovative home care management models. Hopefully, they will learn to capitalize on this important opportunity and share results from more innovative models in the not too distant future.

REFERENCES

Applebaum, R., Seidl, F., & Austin, C. (1980). The Wisconsin Community Care Organization: Preliminary findings from the Milwaukee experiment. *Gerontologist, 20,* 356–63.

Bishop, C., & Skwara, K. C. (1993). Recent growth of Medicare home health. *Health Affairs, 12*(3), 95–110.

Criteria Committee of the New York Heart Association. (1964). *Diseases of the heart and blood vessels.* Boston: Little, Brown.

Cummings, J., Hughes, S. L., & Weaver, F. M. (1992). A multi-site randomized trial of team managed VA hospital based home care. Funded by the Department of Veterans Affairs, Cooperative Centers for Studies in Health Services (#3), 1992–1997.

Cummings, J., Hughes, S. L., Weaver, F. M., Manheim, L., Conrad, K., Nash, K., Braun, B., & Adelman, J. (1990). Cost-effectiveness of V.A. hospital-based home care: A randomized clinical trial. *Archives of Internal Medicine, 150,* 1274–1280.

Gooding, J., & Jette, A. M. (1985). Hospital readmissions among the elderly. *Journal of the American Geriatrics Society, 33,* 595–601.

Hedrick, S. C., & Inui, T. S. (1986). The effectiveness and cost of home care: An information synthesis. *Health Services Research, 20,* 851–879.

Hughes, S. L. (1985). Apples and oranges? A review of demonstrations and evaluations of community-based long term care. *Health Services Research, 20,* 461–488.

———. (1991). Home care: Where we are and where we need to go. In M. G. Ory & A. P. Duncker (Eds.), *In-home care for older people* (pp. 53–74). Newbury Park, CA: Sage.

———. (1992). Services for the continuum—home health. In C. Evashwick (Ed.), *The continuum of long-term care: An integrated systems approach* (pp. 61–79). Albany, NY: Delmar.

Hughes, S. L., Cummings, J., Weaver, F. M., Manheim, L., Braun, B., & Conrad, K. (1992). A randomized trial of the cost-effectiveness of home health care for the terminally ill. *Health Services Research, 26,* 801–817.

Hughes, S. L., Cummings, J., Weaver, F.M., Manheim, L., Conrad, K., & Nash,

K. (1990). A randomized trial of VA home care for severely disabled veterans. *Medical Care, 28,* 135–145.

Kantrowitz, A. (1988). State of the art circulatory support. *Transactions—American Society for Artificial Internal Organs, 34,* 445–449.

Kemper, P. R., Applebaum, R., & Harrigan, M. (1988). Community care demonstrations: What have we learned? *Health Care Financing Review, 8*(4), 87–100.

Kemper, P. R., Brown, R. S., Carcagno, G. J., Applebaum, R. A., Christianson, J. B., Corson, W., Dunstan, S. M., Grannemann, T., Harrigan, M., Holden, N., Phillips, B. R., Schore, J., Thornton, C., Wooldridge, J., & Skidmore, F. (1988). The evaluation of the national long-term care demonstration [Special issue]. *Health Services Research, 23*(1).

Komisar, H. L., & Feder, J. (1998). *The Balanced Budget Act of 1997: Effect on Medicare's home health benefit and beneficiaries who need long-term care.* New York: The Commonwealth Fund.

Montgomery, R., Gonyea, J., & Hooyman, N. (1985). Caregiving and the experience of subjective and objective burden. *Family Relations, 34*(1), 19–26.

Rust, M. E. (1992, July). Home care revival. *American Medical News,* pp. 23–26.

Shaughnessy, P. W., Schlenker, R. E., & Hittle, D. F. (1994). Home health outcomes under captitated and fee-for-service payment. *Health Care Financing Review, 16*(1), 187–222.

U.S. General Accounting Office. (1998). *Medicare home health benefit: Impact of interim payment system and agency closures on access to services* (238GAO/HEHS-98-238). Washington, DC: Author.

Ware, J. E., & Sherbourne, C. D. (1992). The MOS 36–item short-form health survey. *Medical Care, 30,* 473–481.

Weissert, W. G., Cready, C. M., & Pawelak, J. (1988). The past and future of home and community-based long-term care. *Milbank Quarterly, 66,* 309–389.

Welch, H. G., Wennberg, D. E., & Welch, W. P. (1996). The use of Medicare home health care services. *New England Journal of Medicine, 33,* 324–329.

CHAPTER 10

Assuring Quality in Care at Home

Rosalie A. Kane

The rapid growth of home care for people of all ages with chronic illnesses and disabilities intensifies concern about the quality of that care. Preoccupation with quality and quality assurance (QA) programs in home care is, in part, a direct consequence of the growth of public expenditures on home care under Medicare, Medicaid, and state-funded programs. When public entities purchase services rather than deliver them directly (which is the predominant model in health care and long-term care in the United States), public officials require accountability regarding two general issues:

1. Is money being well spent or, conversely, is it being squandered?
2. Does the care provided meet community quality standards? A corollary question here is, Can government officials be sure that the worst case scenario—a care scandal involving death, injury, or abuse—does not occur on their watch?

This chapter examines the range of approaches to QA in home care and considers the extent to which the necessary safeguards against egregious care and the desired incentives toward excellent care and care improvement are in place. First, however, the discussion is put into a context by consideration of the great diversity of in-home programs and the emphasis on home care as an alternative to care somewhere else.

TYPES OF HOME CARE PROGRAMS

Home care tends to be balkanized by the funding streams that support it. The Medicare program, for example, covers home health care for seniors and other beneficiaries who need skilled services and have rehabilitation potential. Medicare also covers hospice services (the vast majority of which are provided in the home) for beneficiaries who are dying and elect the hospice benefit (see chapter 5). Some Medicaid programs and state-funded programs cover ongoing personal care or attendant services to low-income people who need the care, regardless of their rehabilitation potential. Private insurance programs may also cover in-home services; most typically the covered services resemble Medicare home health, but sometimes, particularly for long-term care insurance, a broader range of services may be covered.

Funding programs typically set quality parameters by their definitions of covered services. For example, in some programs a registered nurse must closely supervise activities like catheter care and administration of medications, whereas in other programs (in at least some states), it is acceptable for an attendant with no certification or license to take instructions from the care consumers whose chronic needs are being met, or from their agents. In some real sense, quality in terms of personnel standards and structural criteria are defined specifically by funding program, leading to a great deal of variability across and within states as well as in the way quality is defined for different target clientele. Furthermore, the lengths to which a home care provider is expected to go to achieve rehabilitation results for the patient in the name of quality are both mandated and circumscribed by program features. To illustrate, a vigilant effort to improve upper body motion in a chair-bound or bed-bound consumer with multiple sclerosis may represent a commendable quest for high-quality outcomes, or it may be perceived as a fraudulent use of Medicaid dollars to care for someone without official rehabilitation potential.

HOME CARE QUALITY AND ALTERNATIVES TO HOME CARE

Home care has sometimes been perceived as good in itself in contrast to care in alternative sites such as nursing homes or hospitals. So-called formal home care (i.e., care and help at home from paid professionals and other in-home workers, as distinguished from care and help at home from relatives and friends who are not compensated) has been encouraged and subsidized with the explicit and implicit intention of its being a substitute for more expensive and less user-friendly care in institutions. The chain of reasoning goes as follows: People prefer to live in their own homes rather than in hospitals, nursing homes, and other institutions; home care is less expensive than institutional care; home care prevents or shortens institutional stays; therefore, having home care is a good outcome in terms of the quality of life of consumers and cost. These contentions are at best half-truths. For example, under some conditions and for some conditions, home care may be more expensive than institutional care, the evidence that home care delays or prevents institutional care is scant and contradictory, and, therefore, the cost benefits cannot be relied upon without many caveats.

The arguments about the cost effectiveness of home care as an alternative require clarity about the alternatives. If home care is an alternative to hospital care, home care could reach a high cost and yet be cost effective. In the last 10 years, even ventilator-dependent children formerly cared for in intensive care units receive care at home (Arras, 1995). Less dramatically, home health care has laid claims to shortening or even occasionally preventing hospital care for elderly Medicare beneficiaries. Note, however, that hospital stays under Medicare have already been dramatically shortened as a response to prospective hospital reimbursement for diagnosis-related groups (DRGs); in this milieu, the effect of home care on hospital use might be more subtle and harder to find, perhaps achieved through the route of fewer complications causing rehospitalization.

Home care has also been perceived as an alternative to care in hospitals for persons who have chronic mental illness, and as an alternative to care in various kinds of institutions for people with mental retardation (MR) and developmental disabilities (DD) (e.g., state hospital schools, and MR-DD intermediate care institutions). Advocacy groups for these target populations have, to their credit, been effective in arguing the intrinsic merits of deinstitutionalization and have moved to create a new system without getting mired down in attempts to prove the cost effectiveness of home- and community-based services (HCBS) models compared to the old institutions, which by now have been so radically downsized that their costs per person have been transformed. The downside of this advocacy is that few data are available to examine cost-effectiveness. We know that the costs per capita under the home- and community-based Medicaid waivers specific to MR-DD are very high, and that over 80% of all dollars spent on HCBS waiver programs in 1992 went for MR-DD waivers. On a more positive note, innovative programs for people with disability in which consumers and/or their agents tailor their own care and draw down from a budget to pay for it have shown that MR-DD expenditures need not be astronomical—and, moreover, will better conform to consumer preferences than programs designed by professionals (Nerney & Shumway, 1996).

For older people, home care is often viewed as an alternative to nursing home care. Numerous HCBS experiments and demonstrations over the last two decades were fueled by the idea that timely and appropriate service at home could prevent or delay nursing home admissions that are so costly for societal and family budgets and so dreaded by the populace. The quest for alternatives to nursing homes has a mixed history. Some well-designed and closely watched demonstrations seemed to show that home care was *not* cost effective compared to nursing homes (Carcagno & Kemper, 1988). This body of research has in turn been critiqued and its external generalizability questioned (Kane, 1988; Weissert, 1988; Wiener & Harris, 1990). Among the criticisms: (1) even when the clientele enrolled were very disabled and sick, the demonstrations often failed to find groups likely to enter nursing homes or, if entering, likely to stay there long; (2) the mix of services offered were insufficiently medically oriented to provide the key nursing and health-related services needed to keep people out of nursing homes; and (3) the pricing of in-home services was too high and the level of personnel too professionalized to compete with the bundled and discounted price of a nursing-home day under Medicaid in most states.

The last two points seem contradictory: on the one hand, health-oriented home care as well as in-home personal care and housekeeping services are needed if home care is to be a genuine alternative to nursing homes, and on the other hand, we need to find a way to make such services less expensive in their unit costs and perhaps less professionally dominated, which mitigates against health-oriented care. This poses a challenge for QA in home care, namely, to restructure the delivery system to render it less professionally orthodox at the very same time as we try to improve its capability to provide *health* care and *health* monitoring. Otherwise, state efforts to change their long-term care allocations so that they are less a lopsided subsidy of nursing homes (Kane, Kane, Ladd, & Veazie, 1998; Ladd, Kane, Kane, & Neilsen, 1995) are likely to fail because of the high costs of care at home. Some people would argue that the essence of quality in home care is that in-home services be available in sufficient volume to permit people to stay in least restrictive (or, in newer terminology, most integrated) settings.

The point that people desire to stay at home and fear entering institutions (especially long-stay institutions) is almost indisputably correct, but we are entering into an era of some confusion about what counts as "home" and what is the purview of a home health agency (Kane, 1995a). Home care is no longer easily defined as a service for the homebound; arguably the goals of home care and personal assistant services encompass whatever assistance is needed for the consumers to conduct their ordinary lives. Depending on age and social roles, care may need to be available at schools, workplaces, and places of recreation, and, indeed, home care workers increasingly accompany their clients out of their homes. Also, the face of what used to be known as "institutional" care is changing. More and more, residential care settings are construed along a social model in adult foster care, small group homes, and assisted living setting. At one extreme, assisted living facilities (ALFs) offer apartment-style living where the tenants—also needful of care—live lives where privacy, dignity, choice, individualization, and opportunity for normal lifestyles are maximized (Kane & Wilson, 1993). If ALF staff render care to residents in their own apartments according to individual care plans and consumer preferences, this somewhat resembles home care. If, as often happens, home health agencies provide care to residents of ALFs and other kinds of LTC settings, boundaries are more definitely blurred, resulting in some confusion over who is in charge of the case.

Although some might still judge the quality of home care by its cost effectiveness as an alternative to something else, the rest of this chapter ignores that issue. Rather, it focuses on the quality of home care per se and the search for sensible public policies to ensure or improve that quality.

QA TECHNOLOGY AND HOME CARE

The QA Cycle

QA has become a field (as well as a growth industry), in itself, and is replete with jargon. But, when stripped to its essentials, the steps of quality assurance for any health care endeavor are logical and straightforward. Any QA cycle has three general steps: (1) defining quality by establishing criteria and standards by which quality will be judged; (2) inspecting or assessing the care to determine whether the standards were met; and (3) correcting any identified problem, and preventing its recurrence. Each part of this cycle is difficult to accomplish, and the first two steps seem futile without the third.

Quality Definition

The first step—defining quality—is sometimes separated into structure, process, and outcome. Structural criteria refer to those elements of the program (e.g., staff qualifications, management practices, equipment, record keeping, appeals processes) thought to be necessary to ensure adequate care. Process criteria refer to the procedures followed in particular cases and for people with particular conditions. The processes desired may be general (e.g., infection control procedures) or specific to managing a disease (e.g., diabetes) or a treatment (e.g., administration of IV antibiotics). Outcome criteria refer to the results of care (e.g., extent of disability, pain and pain relief, health status, health complications, psychological status, or social well-being).

Standard setting for home care is made more complicated by the variety of goals and programs encompassed in home care. Home care encompasses the highest of technology and the lowest. It embraces Medicare home health, hospice, a variety of Medicaid-funded home care and personal assistant services (PAS) programs (also called personal attendant services), and respite care. Its goals may include specific rehabilitation objectives (e.g., ambulation, speech, or bladder control); preventing complications of illnesses, producing patients and families able to care for themselves, longer lives, comfortable deaths, and reduced "unmet need." When the home care consumers have chronic and perhaps permanent disabling conditions, then the home care providers must incorporate as a major goal that the consumers perceive their lives as productive and meaningful.

A growing body of literature has emerged about what home care clients actually value. Summarizing this work (some resulting from focus groups and some from surveys) leads to the conclusion that, although technical competence with health care is important and expected, consumers' endorsements hinge as much on other attributes. Most often mentioned are reliability (e.g., honesty, trustworthiness, showing up on time), kindness and courtesy, compatibility, and genuine caring and concern. These qualities are not embodied in the kind of process criteria that examine technical aspects of care (Was the bed made properly? Was the medication administered correctly?). In an earlier work on quality in home care, we proposed the term *enabling criteria* for these rather obvious and necessary features of a high-quality home care provider, such as honesty, courtesy, timeliness, and dependability (Kane, Kane, Illston, & Eustis, 1994).

Quality Assessment

The second step—assessing quality—requires other detailed decisions. Who should do this assessment? When? How often? What evidence will be considered accurate? Should the assessment be based on samples of consumers or other observers of care? Should the approach be one of encouraging and vigorously investigating complaints, or should care be monitored routinely on some kind of sampling basis?

The home is often contrasted with more controlled health care settings (hospitals, nursing homes, even ambulatory clinics) where the encounters between health care providers and consumers are more visible and easily tracked. The private home is just that—*private.* The encounters between home care workers and their clientele are not readily observed. Moreover, for some aspects of home care, particularly the relationship with the in-home workers, only the consumer will be able to adequately judge whether quality has been adequate. Other safeguards besides consumer opinion are needed to monitor technical aspects of home care, but some information must come directly from home care consumers or their agents. This need introduces strategic questions about how to overcome the well-known reluctance of older consumers to criticize a service upon which they depend.

Continuous Quality Improvement

The three-part cycle of QA just described applies to QA activities external to the home care provider (e.g., governmental inspectors or accrediting bodies) or to activities undertaken by the agencies themselves to monitor and upgrade the care they provide. The latter activities, highly favored in the 1990s, are often called continuous quality improvement (CQI) or total quality management (TQM). In a CQI effort, the energy and creativity of the entire work, especially its units closest to the consumer and the production of service, are engaged in identifying and defining problems and reaching solutions. However, any CQI effort must be informed by a data base or information system describing care and its results, and must be capable of determining whether care is, in fact, improving, according to some objective criteria.

GOOD QA PRACTICES

Criteria to evaluate home care are not identical to criteria to evaluate QA efforts in home care (Kane, Frytak, Thomas, & Eustis, 1995). Indeed, it is a long-standing problem related to QA in any sector to decide whether identification of numerous problems means that a QA system is working well or poorly. One would ideally like a QA system to act to prevent problems. On the other hand, one would like a QA system to be able to identify any problems that were occurring. Despite these caveats, if QA efforts were functioning properly, in a general way, we would expect the following:

- The overall quality of care be high.
- *Important* problems are readily identified.
- Identified problems are promptly corrected.
- The same kind of quality problems do not keep recurring.
- Consumers have confidence in the care.
- Consumers initiate complaints about poor quality.
- The QA system has positive incentives to improve performance and no negative incentives.
- Information is generated that allows the quality of care to be compared according to consumer characteristics and according to providers;
- The burden of the QA program for consumers and providers is low and the overall cost of the program is as low as possible.
- The QA program offers due process protections to agencies and individuals alleged to be performing poorly (as far as is consistent with protecting consumers).

Note that these criteria are neutral as to the actual definition of quality, which could emphasize physical or social well-being, or both, and could rely on structure and process criteria or outcome criteria. But, however quality is defined, the good QA system will identify problems promptly and will concentrate on those problems that have meaning for people's well-being rather than trivial variations from rules that may be easy to measure. The burdens and costs of the QA effort should be minimized (because money spent on QA cannot be spent on services), but these efficiency criteria are secondary to criteria for effectiveness. Also, it is important that the rights of workers be protected in a QA system, but these rights should not take precedence over the rights of vulnerable consumers.

GENERAL QA APPROACHES

QA efforts and programs can be pitched at several levels. Here let us consider five interrelated approaches: regulatory, consumer-oriented, and market or systemic approaches, educational approaches, and provider-initiated approaches. All of these function simultaneously in home care in the United States today, though all have imperfections. The various methods reviewed have different likelihoods of meeting the criteria for a QA system discussed above. In developing the proper blend of approaches, one is also forced to consider who bears responsibility for the quality of home care.

Regulatory Approaches

The most commonly considered QA approach is regulatory. Governments attempt to influence quality by establishing licensing programs for individual professionals and for agencies. Thus, the quality of home care is potentially influenced by a state's requirements for agencies doing home care in its jurisdiction, and also by rules defining professional practices such as nursing or physical therapy. If certain practices are defined as nursing and forbidden to personnel without a nursing license, then paraprofessionals cannot do the service at all. Some argue that such restrictions protect all consumers and improve quality overall; others argue that restriction of certain practices such as administering medications, catheter care, wound care, and so on to licensed nurses makes home care too costly for many privately paying people and encourages provision of these kinds of care by unlicensed people without any oversight at all. In contrast, some states have widely expanded the potential for nurses to teach unlicensed personnel how to do nursing procedures and do not view home care as a service that must usually be closely supervised by a nurse. A recent thorough evaluation mandated by the state of Washington in connection with new, somewhat permissive, nurse practice legislation was unable to detect any quality problems caused by the changed standard (Young & Sikma, 1998).

In addition to governmental licensure authority, public bodies can and do inspect the care that they finance. Inspections of home care have been somewhat perfunctory compared to the attention given to nursing homes. Federal inspections for home health care under Medicare are especially unexacting. Home health agencies are deemed to meet federal standards if they are accredited by the National League of Nursing or the Joint Commission on Accreditation of Health Care Organizations. Since the mid-1990s, Medicare Home Health has come under scrutiny because of its rapid growth, and some evidence has been found for fraudulent billings and other abuses (US. General Accounting Office, 1995, 1997, 1998); however, the focus of these inquiries has been on the need for and appropriateness of expenditures rather than the actual quality of care.

One reason why state-funded and -managed home care has not been inspected vigorously by governmental regulators is the absence of agreed-upon methods. Over the last decade, however, states have made substantial progress in determining how they will define and monitor quality of home care and PAS under their Medicaid, Medicaid-waiver, and state-funded programs. Some states, such as South Carolina (Geron & Kane, 1991), Wisconsin (The Management Group, 1995), Ohio (Applebaum & McGinnis, 1992), and Indiana (Kinney, Friedman, & Loveland Cook, 1994), to name a few, have developed protocols to monitor the quality of home care in ways that include both record audits and actual contact with consumers.

States sometimes require that personnel receive criminal checks before they can work in a client's home. States vary in who must have such checks (paraprofessional personnel only or all personnel; personnel employed by agencies, independently employed workers, or both) and who bears the cost for the criminal check (the state or county, an employing agency as part of its licensing requirements, or the clients).

Consumer Centered Approaches

To complement or even to obviate regulatory approaches, some would argue that consumers need assistance to become much more directly engaged in seeking quality in their home care and to complain about poor-quality care. With that in mind, 1987 federal legislation required hotlines for complaints about home care; however, these lines are seldom used. In some jurisdictions, the long-term care ombudsman program, which has a statutory responsibility to mediate problems and resolve complaints in nursing homes and board-and-care homes, has moved into the home care arena. However, the system of regular visitation established for facilities does not lend itself to home care, and in most areas the ombudsman program barely has resources to deal with its official mandate (Harris-Wehling, Feasley, & Estes, 1995).

Other consumer-oriented activities include consumer watchdog groups, rating systems and report cards done by independent programs, consumer education strategies, and consumer empowerment strategies. To the extent that some of these approaches are buttressed by regulated consumer rights or are embodied in licensure requirements, they are closely aligned with regulation. For example, agencies may be required to institute complaint mechanisms, disclose information to consumers, or appoint consumer advisory boards. Some consumer-oriented activities are geared to assist consumers who go outside established agencies to hire their own personnel. Most of the materials have been prepared for younger people with disabilities, but Susik (1995) has prepared a practical guide directed at people in their 70s, 80s, and 90s who choose to hire their own home caregivers.

Market/Systemic Approaches

States or, more usually, counties and municipalities using state dollars are large purchasers of home care. One form of QA is to insert quality requirements into the criteria for bidders or, even better, to undertake competitive bidding on the basis of quality as well as price. At an extreme, advocates of vouchers would argue that this approach would allow the market to operate in upgrading quality. However, in the absence of a vigorous effort to inform consumers as discussed in the preceding section, this strategy seems unpromising.

Without relying on market forces, one can, nonetheless, take a systemic approach to QA for home care in a state or geographic area. Case management, external to home care providers, can be seen as a deliberate mechanism for improving quality, and perhaps even obviating the need for inflexible regulations. Case managers typically have responsibility for assessing need for care, making a care plan in conjunction with the client and with respect for client preferences, purchasing services or making referrals to implement that plan, and monitoring the adequacy of service providers and the well-being of clients. This role would seem to provide a good framework for monitoring quality, and would allow for examining the overall quality of home care from a variety of agency and independently employed providers (Kane & Degenholtz, 1997a). If the state uses a common assessment tool and invests in an information system, a QA system centered on such case management agencies would provide even greater accountability. Furthermore, to the extent that case managers can correct problems by working with vendors or terminating relationships with vendors, they are well positioned to implement the entire QA cycle.

Case managers are not uniformly equipped for QA roles, however. Some programs are structured so that large caseloads prohibit individualization, and some case management programs sharply constrain the extent to which a case manager may work directly with vendors or help clients change vendors. In some instances, case managers may be fixated on controlling public expenditures. Also at issue is whether case managers themselves have the training and skills needed to serve as QA agents. If case managers are to have a major role in assuring the quality of the services they purchase or arrange, a fundamental question is, What assurance is there about the quality of the case managers themselves? Finally, the relationship between case managers and care-providing agencies can become contentious, with the latter asserting that case managers are at best superfluous and at worst intrusive and detrimental to care. The more professionalized and specialized the provider agency, the more the external case management is resented, although clear role delineation can eliminate disagreements (Kane & Frytak, 1994).

Educational Approaches

Professional education and, even more, education of paraprofessional frontline workers is often posited as a critical feature in QA, both to prevent problems in the first place and to remedy identified care plans.

To some extent, this approach is subsumed in regulatory approaches. For example, federal and state regulations and private accreditations typically require that professional personnel have specific minimum credentials and that paraprofessional personnel have specific amounts of preemployment training and that all staff participate in regular staff development sessions. We focus on training for special consideration (as distinct from education) because critics of home care quality place special stock in mandated training. We need to distinguish between basic education in degree-bearing programs from on-the-job training (whether in the form of preemployment training, orientation, or staff development). It may be important to modify the basic education of nurses or other home care professionals to enhance their skills for home care, but this strategy is too slow and uncertain to be major plank in QA.

It is almost an article of faith that paraprofessionals need more training for hands-on home care roles (or for that matter, any hands-on long-term care). Suggested areas for training include skill performance (e.g., transferring, hygiene, assistance with medication administration), knowledge about specific diseases (e.g., Alzheimer's disease, COPD, congestive heart failure) and procedures (e.g., catheter care, ostomy care), and understanding of communication, relationship-building, observational skills, conflict resolution, and the like. Unfortunately, no data are available to show that training leads to better care processes or outcomes. Some hopes for preemployment training seem overly optimistic. It is as if 90 or 120 hours of preemployment training might inoculate the trained worker from all the negative effects exerted on performance by poor working conditions, poor pay, unclear job descriptions, inaccessible supervisors, and unclear lines of authority.

Provider-initiated Efforts

The widespread interest in CQI, mentioned above, is fueled, in part, by a belief that provider-initiated QA has the advantage of providing an active approach to identifying and addressing quality problems rapidly. Regulatory efforts have the disadvantage of being reactive, entailing the identification of problems or patterns of problems after their occurrence. They are often minimalist in terms of frequency, sample size, and depth of surveys. In contrast, efforts initiated by the providers themselves have the advantage of providing a positive approach to overall quality upgrading (not merely eliminating egregious problems) and a potential for rapid correction. Providers have the potential to build quality controls into their standard operating practices, based on good management information systems. Programs designed by particular agencies are often innovative and creative. They cannot replace regulatory and other approaches because of overall governmental responsibility for protection of citizens and responsible expenditures of tax dollars. Yet, if governments and the public had confidence in providers' efforts, they could design their own oversight accordingly. Of course, when care is provided by individually employed workers without agency affiliation, some other technique is needed, which may include a blend of case management oversight, regulatory oversight, and consumer-centered approaches.

QA Strategies for Agencies

Conceptually, we can identify a range of QA approaches open to home care agencies. Some of these are closely tied to the process of delivering care and others are more removed from care delivery. A review of best practices in provider-initiated QA (Kane et al., 1995) developed a classification of strategies used by 128 home care agencies with exemplary QA practices. These 128 were selected by screening from 2,950 home care agencies that responded to a survey inviting all home care agencies to describe QA practices that they viewed as innovative and/or effective.

The categories of QA derived were (1) audits of care for active or closed cases; (2) systematic feedback from consumers (elicited in person, by phone, or by mail); (3) client complain mechanisms; (4) staff training, orientation, and development; (5) supervision and performance evaluation (which could include innovative efforts to make on-site evaluations of worker performance); (6) staff feedback mechanisms, such as case conferences and solicitation of staff feedback (including formal CQI efforts that often entail multiple work groups, and with work groups and widespread staff involvement); (7) specialized recruitment and retention efforts; (8) staff recognition and quality incentives; and (9) innovative care restructuring.

The last category was used to describe a wide range of changes that agencies developed in response to perceived quality challenges. These strategies vary considerably, for example, (1) informal written "contracts" among client, in-home aide, and nurse supervisor during the first visit; (2) a notebook left in the client's home as a "communication center," to which all in-home staff contribute and which can be read by external case managers, clients, and family members; (3) special home health aide progress notes; (4) supportive techniques and buddy systems to work with difficult clients; (5) preprinted charts, care plans, and flow sheets; (6) development and application of high-risk indicators and provision of special care coordination to those at risk; (7) special follow-up efforts with cases that have been closed; and (8) various innovative team and supervisory approaches that modify the roles of nurses and paraprofessional workers. No agency in our sample, however, had truly developed a system to track outcomes for its clientele over time.

Variation in Provider QA

Not surprisingly, given certification requirements, Medicare-certified home health agencies tended to have more elaborate and fully articulated QA strategies than uncertified agencies. Also expectedly, larger agencies and agencies with multiple branch offices were more likely to employ dedicated QA staff. Each QA strategy also had multiple variations. For example, the audits differed not only in frequency, sampling strategies, and modes of data collection, but also by whether it was possible to use the audit data to improve care, which in turn required waiving anonymity.

Relationship to Corrective Action

The extent to which any QA effort actually is used to improve care is unclear. In our study of best practices, we asked agency informants how they would typically identify and correct problems. We used scenarios to hold constant a number of problems ranging from poor relationships between client and worker, no-shows, substandard care, or newly emerging client problems needing attention (e.g., depression). Agencies varied widely in the extent to which their own identified QA strategies were seen by them as relevant to identifying and correcting problems (Kane, Frytak, & Eustis, 1997).

UNRESOLVED ISSUES

Defining a Cohesive Strategy at the State Level

State governments have at their disposal a wide variety of direct and indirect ways of having an impact on the quality of home care, using the full range of activities described above. The most direct vehicles include (1) standard-setting through licensure of provider organizations, (2) standard-setting through licensure or certification of home care personnel, including paraprofessionals, (3) standard-setting through requirements for vendors under Medicaid and other state-funded programs, (4) inspection and monitoring of licensed entities or personnel funded through state programs, and (5) corrective action and sanctions at the state level (fines, delicensing, withdrawal of vendor status, criminal sanctions).

At their discretion, states can create other programs to influence the quality of home care. For example, the case management (also known as care coordination) programs that states develop for home care can be deliberately designed to provide accountability for the allocation of in-home services and their quality. The long-term care ombudsman program, which has a statutory responsibility (under the Older Americans Act) for mediation and complaint resolution for Medicaid nursing home and board-and-care-home clientele, can be expanded to include home care. States can allocate funds to create registries of home care employees, to perform criminal checks for some or all people working in the home setting, or to develop curricula or conduct state-level training for home care personnel. Complementing regulatory efforts, states also can build on procedural and structural requirements by developing and disseminating educational material for consumers and providers.

Without necessarily expanding funds to operate QA programs directly, state governments can influence the nature and quality of home care through enunciating principles in statute (e.g., a home care bill of rights, a philosophy of care) or enacting requirements for QA (e.g., paraprofessional training, criminal checks, QA procedures, and reporting procedures) that are passed on to home care agencies as conditions of being licensed to become a vendor for a funded program.

Reaching a desirable blend of public policies calls for consideration of how, if at all, home care differs from other care with respect to QA challenges—the goals expected from home care and the extent to which home care quality is actually a problem, as well as the nature of that problem. Below are issues that need attention for attaining a desirable blend.

Accountability for Home Care Quality

Arguably, home care poses particular challenges because the home is the domain of client and family rather than the workplace of health care providers. Clients can and do call the shots about what happens in the home. Providers have sometimes used this fact as an argument for their having only limited accountability for the outcomes of their efforts. Furthermore, family members play ambiguous roles in home care. Sometimes they are perceived as objects of a home care plan (i.e., the goal is to relieve family burdens or to train family caregivers). Sometimes they seem to be adjuncts of a home care plan (i.e., family members are caregivers, who must meet measurable quality standards). And sometimes they are viewed as contextual players who interfere with the provider's efforts to provide quality care and achieve desirable outcomes.

In addition, scrutiny of home care is difficult, because the care occurs in individual dwellings and includes numerous unobserved encounters. This might argue for attention to measurable outcomes, which can be expressed in terms of averages rather than detailed attention to process and structure. However, many providers are reluctant to take on even limited responsibility for outcomes other than rather narrow ones—for example, improved knowledge by consumers of their own health status and functional conditions (Kane et al., 1994).

Getting Agreement on Goals

Home care is, of course, a varied phenomenon. In general, however, the goals for most home care consumers will include a mixture of therapeutic goals (e.g., measurable improvement or decline in rate of deterioration on specified functions or health indicators) and goals that have no relationship to therapy or rehabilitation in the conventional sense of the terms, such as those that improve or maintain the consumer's quality of life. The bleak and dispiriting term *custodial care* has sometimes been used for care at home or in facilities if that care fails to strive to improve some health or functional parameter. This is an unfortunate term, however, because the meeting of residual care needs (i.e., needs that cannot be met by use of specialized equipment but rather require human assistance) can be done in a way that enhances or diminishes the consumer's quality of life, and the very term *custodial* (usually associated with jail custody) suggests that custodial approaches will diminish rather than enhance life.

The way everyday care at home is detailed into tasks, timed, and carried out can influence that consumer's family life, social life, ordinary activities, sense of autonomy, and social well-being. Elsewhere, I have suggested that the term *compensatory goals* might be a better to refer to care that is meant to compensate for impairments that are stable and are unlikely to improve (Kane, 1999). Specifying the improvements expected from compensatory care in narrow clinical terms would involve considerable hubris and, arguably, misplaced energy, even though the purpose of the care is to enable consumers to live as full a life as possible given the impairment. The consumer is, perhaps, the only person who can indicate the extent to which compensatory care is of fully adequate quality. Yet assessment by the consumer, though necessary, is insufficient to gauge the quality of care that is technical in nature. Technical attributes are often relevant to care regardless of whether goals are therapeutic or compensatory, and indeed consumers care about *both* kinds of goals. A mixed strategy for improving accountability will be necessary, including both the subjectivity of the consumer and some technical standards developed by professionals. The relative emphasis surely should depend on the nature of the service delivered and the cognitive capacity of the consumer.

Goal conflict is likely to occur in home care, requiring decisions about whose goals take priority and how such conflicts are resolved. We know that different stake holders in the home care process (consumers, families, providers, payers, and regulators) prioritize goals differently and also have different preferences for outcomes versus process as criteria for meeting the goals (Kane et al., 1994). If safety is held as the most important goal, and a large list of process and structure criteria associated with safety mirror professional orthodoxy, it is likely that the costs of care will rise and client preferences will take second place to professional views. Very little research is available to assess providers' or case managers' knowledge of these values. Some preliminary research suggests that consumers vary markedly in what they hold important and even in how they define values such as safety and privacy, as well as the characteristics they would most seek in a person providing them with help in their homes (Degenholtz, Kane, & Kivnick, 1997; Kane, 1995b; Kane & Degenholtz, 1997b).

Improving Measures

Once the decision is made to get data directly from consumers, one must overcome technical problems. These include the well-known reluctance of many older people to criticize those providing care, both because of inherent courtesy and because of dependence on providers. In an innovative computer-assisted quality assurance program in Indiana (Kinney et al., 1994), clients were asked to rate the quality of care of each in-home provider and were also given an open-ended opportunity to comment on things they would like to have different. The ratings generally were very positive, yet the comments mentioned tardiness, theft, anxiety over children brought along or left in cars, and disturbing smoking on the job.

Obviously, great attention must be given to who requests feedback and how the request is couched. In addition, it would be convenient to have standardized instruments available to capture quality along the dimensions deemed important to consumers. Several projects are under way to develop measures to tap consumers perceptions of the quality of in-home services. One of the most carefully developed and furthest along was designed by Geron (1997) as part of a National Institute of Aging project. The resultant Home Care Satisfaction Measures (HCRI) taps the following dimensions viewed by clients as important: provider competency, system adequacy, positive interpersonal items, and negative interpersonal items. Other researchers have attempted to measure "unmet need" as a way to tap the quality of home care, for example, for each functional impairment. Allen and Mor (1997) measured the difficulty the respondent has in doing the activity without help and the presence of one or more bad consequences that might be a proxy for inadequacy of help. Capitman, Abrahams, and Ritter (1997) similarly measured the consequences of inadequate amounts of care as one domain of quality; they also demonstrated some success in measuring quality through telephone interviews with consumers.

In a different vein, with funding from the HCFA, Shaughnessy and colleagues have developed the OASIS, a monitoring system for home health quality based on a standardized national assessment (Shaughnessy et al., 1994; see also chapter 8).

Reactions to Bad Outcomes for Home Care Clients

With home care, as with other LTC services, rhetoric of providers, regulators, consumer advocates, and policymakers tends to encourage consumer autonomy, normal lifestyles, and the right to take informed risks. However, home care providers tend to feel responsible when anything bad happens to someone under their care, for example, falls, relapses, victimization, or other mishaps. More societal dialogue is necessary about the extent of the responsibility of home care providers for anything that happens to clients under their care, especially since similar bad events overtake vulnerable elderly people living in their own homes without home care. The special situations involving Alzheimer's disease and other dementias need attention because the extent to which family members and guardians should be responsible for making decisions involving risk is a gray area of practice and of law. Overall, it is necessary to consider, perhaps with use of case examples, how to differentiate between true neglect or dereliction of duty and calculated risks gone wrong. Finally, we need a range of approaches to make mid-course corrections in programs, in order to minimize all bad results, while avoiding overreaction that cuts off opportunities for the majority of clients to live meaningful lives at home. Certainly the bulk of ethical dilemmas that arise for home care practitioners concern this very issue of how to make tradeoffs between freedom and preferences of the consumer, on the one hand, and a view of consumer safety, on the other (Kane & Caplan, 1993).

How Good or Bad Is Home Care?

It is startling that, in fact, we have little information about the extent to which a quality problem exists in home care. There is a general belief that as home care increases, quality problems will also increase. As yet, however, there is no evidence of widespread problems in the quality of home care.

There is some evidence that access to both home health care and socially oriented home care is insufficient under various circumstances. For example, Shaughnessy, Schlenker, and Hittle (1994) suggest that Medicare beneficiaries receive less home health care and experience more complications if they are in HMOs as opposed to fee for service. And the presence of waiting lists for state in-home services programs suggests that there is not enough funding to meet all the identifiable need. But, despite anxiety-raising reports in the popular press chronicling instances of criminals working in home care (Eisler, 1996), no systematic data are available to indicate whether a systemic problem exists. In the home health arena, as stated above, there is much more evidence of business fraud and abuse of programmatic rules than there is evidence of poor quality. And in the area of non-Medicare home care, most of the expressed problems concern insufficient amounts of service and inflexibility in service provision rather than poor quality of actual procedures or outcomes. Most definitely, the information base about in-home services under Medicaid waivers and state programs is skimpy, however, leading to debates about whether the "no news" about large problems in home care should be considered reassuring.

FUTURE AGENDA

This chapter concludes with suggestions for an agenda related to home care QA, including conceptual and theoretical needs and fruitful future research.*

Conceptual Challenges

Conceptual challenges can be posed as a series of questions:

1. Should home care quality be measured by absence of negative events and conditions, and/or by positive features of good care (outcome and process)? Related to this:
   a. To what extent should the goals of home care be considered therapeutic (e.g., measured in improvements or stabilization of conditions and functional abilities), and to what extent should they be considered compensatory for functional impairments (e.g., measured by ability of people to lead somewhat normal lives)?
   b. For therapeutic goals, should maintenance of function be separated from improvement of function?
   c. What balance between outcome and process indicators is desirable, and why?
2. To what extent is quality of home care fairly judged by quality of life measures?
   a. Should home care providers be expected to time and arrange care in such a way as to maximize preferred social activities of consumers?
   b. Is the quality of interaction between home care providers and consumers important to the quality of life construct?

---

*This section is adapted and updated from the results of a working conference to create a research and demonstration agenda related to quality assurance and quality improvement held in Baltimore on August 29, 1995, as part of a Health Care Financing Administration grant to the University of Minnesota to conduct studies in the quality of home care, Robert L. Kane (P.I.).

c. Is home care somehow different from other forms of long-term care in relation to quality of life concerns, and, if so, why?
d. How much weight should be given to consumer satisfaction, consumer perception of convenience of service, and other aspects of consumer satisfaction?
3. How should technical and more general aspects of quality be incorporated into a quality assurance system, including
a. aspects of quality, if any, that are beyond the capacity of the consumers to judge?
b. aspects of quality, if any, that can be judged *only* by consumer reactions? Should a quality agenda include a determination of how to achieve adequate or excellent quality at lower prices? Given a willingness to spend the same aggregate dollars on home care, and if we assume an inverse relationship between unit price of home care and amount of care given to an individual or a community group, then, arguably, one dimension of quality—individual and/or population access to care—goes up as price goes down.
5. How does one distinguish operationally between unmet need for home care and independence? Are existing ADL measures sufficiently sensitive to measure unmet need, on the one hand, and independent functioning, on the other?

Research Questions

Answers to the following questions would be useful to guide home care QA efforts:
1. What is known about the prevalence of quality problems in home care, including home health care, personal care, and socially oriented home care?
2. What client factors describe the amount, type, and auspice of home care received, and what difference does this make? Surprisingly little is known about how home care gets allocated. For seniors in managed care organizations, there is not even a workable typology of the different kind of arrangements for the allocation of home care, which could be done under various kinds of direct provisions or contracts with varying kinds of financial incentives.
3. What, if any, types of quality problems are of greatest concern? Are such problems largely technical, relational, or both?

Assuring Quality in Care at Home

4. How do quality problems vary according to characteristics of clients, characteristics of providers, and specific payment programs?
5. Do we have any evidence supporting various structural and procedural standards for home care quality (e.g., credentials, preemployment training, supervisory levels)?
6. From various perspectives (e.g., providers, regulators, state and federal officials), what are the next important, unanswered questions about home care quality where results might suggest changes in practice or policy?

Possible Demonstration Projects or Major Initiatives

1. The relative merits of external versus internal (i.e., provider-based) case management could be studied through demonstration projects. Options include
   a. a relatively narrow study related to home health or a broader study
   b. an examination of how a structured approach to QA housed in a case management program (e.g., with standards, assessment tools, etc.) compares with a standard case management program or no case management
   c. an investigation of whether case management as QA has greater payoff when care is not provided by the agencies doing case management
2. The effectiveness of consumer-based QA efforts could be examined, including:
   a. the effects of vouchers or cash to consumers to purchase care under various rules (e.g., comparing unconstrained consumer choice to caveats about who can do what)
   b. the relative effectiveness of using different approaches to empower and inform consumers
   c. the characteristics of consumers who can participate in consumer-based programs and the effectiveness of family proxies in these roles when consumers are cognitively impaired.
3. Demonstration of personnel policies/substitutions would be helpful, including
   a. projects geared to show what kinds of personnel arrangements are consistent with quality processes and outcomes
   b. demonstrations to show whether consumers are better or worse

off, and in what ways, when higher paid personnel are replaced wholly or in part by less expensive personnel
   c. demonstrations to inform the effects of using less intensive supervision in home care on access to home care. Better access could be defined as both more units of service per person for same cost, or more coverage of unmet need in catchment area
4. Related to the above, demonstrations of downward delegation by nurses of nursing services in home care settings would be timely. Such studies could examine both delegation to unlicensed home care workers and formal delegation to family members. These could inform policy issues such as desirable standards surrounding delegation, the desirable discretion for nurses when providing technical assistance, and the most effective payment and reporting mechanisms.
5. Outcomes-based quality demonstration could examine the effectiveness of various agency strategies. Among the possible variations, the demonstrations could
   a. follow specific conditions at agency level, with the agency determining its own QA mechanisms if quality benchmarks are met
   b. develop and test a strategy for providers to track a small number of parameters on individual patients that serve as a trigger mechanisms for an intervention if preset goals for each parameter are not met in a given time frame
   c. use case mix–adjusted quality of care and/or quality of life measures to identify good providers, both for consumer report cards and regulation
6. Demonstrations could shed light on utilization of technology and management information systems (MIS) to get consumers involved in care and to help them provide feedback to providers. It would be feasible to test MIS at the agency level, which in turn feeds MIS at the systems level, and to develop and test ways for consumers to provide information at the end of each encounter that is incorporated into MIS.
7. One could systematically demonstrate the effects of changing various licensing and structural standards. For example, one could
   a. evaluate the effectiveness of licensing home care agencies based on their performance, removing structural criteria for persons employed by that agency

b. test the relative contribution of preemployment training and requirements for credentials versus various ways that work is structured, supervised, and reimbursed
8. Demonstrations and research projects could be designed to explore what contributes to the quality of the paraprofessional labor force. For example, one could
   a. study which contributes most to quality—the amount paraprofessionals are paid or the amount of oversight and training they get
   b. examine the extent to which acceptable quality personnel are available in various markets and how to alleviate shortages (e.g., how increased payment and benefits for paraprofessionals influences labor supply)
   c. examine whether retention of workers is a necessary or important strategy for labor force development or whether planned short-term labor (new high school and college graduates) could achieve quality results
   d. develop and test supervisory models (e.g., looking at the use of technology such as bar-coded record keeping or computers to better monitor the care given by paraprofessionals)
9. External advocacy and complaint-resolution efforts could be studied to ask questions such as
   a. To what extent does creation of advocacy mechanisms result in quality problems coming to the attention of providers and regulators in a timely way?
   b. What predicts consumer use of complaint/advocacy mechanisms?
   c. How can advocates and hotlines be effectively publicized and organized?
10. For people who are dually eligible for Medicare and Medicaid, one could test different relationships between home health and socially oriented care, including different ways of making capitation payments. For example, a demonstration could compare the effects for different subgroups of capitations to socially oriented agencies, which then purchase nursing services, versus care capitated to health agencies that purchase personal care and homemaking on an "as needed" basis.
11. Studies are needed to develop QA technology itself. Particularly needed are
    a. measures of consumer satisfaction

b. measures of extent to which new health conditions or functional decline is noted by home care providers
   c. development of optimal data collection and sampling strategies

This is an ambitious research agenda that is unlikely to be fully accomplished. Yet illustrative studies are already under way or complete that address various parts of the agenda, including consumer empowerment through cash payments or vouchers (Mahoney & Simon-Rusinowitz, 1997), comparison of consumer-directed care with agency care (Benjamin et. al, 1998), delegation of nursing function (Young & Sikma, 1998), and development of measures and other QA technology.

With no claim to being comprehensive, the diversity of this agenda is noteworthy. Its breadth stems from the variety of QA approaches possible, as discussed in this chapter. The agenda is also born, in part, out of skepticism about many things taken for granted—from the importance of training to the negative effects of high staff turnover. Very little can now be taken as given. Whatever research is done, however, it would seem important to keep in mind several overriding principles: that consumers should be at the center of the QA process, that neither a social nor a medical model is sufficient, and that QA efforts should be designed so that existing practices can be modified and innovation in home care can occur.

REFERENCES

Allen, S. M. & Mor, V. (1997). The prevalence and consequences of unmet need. *Medical Care, 35*(11), 101–172.

Applebaum, R. A., & McGinnis, R. (1992). What price quality? Assuring the quality of case-managed in-home care. *Journal of Case Management, 1*(2), 9–13.

Arras, J. (Ed). (1995*). Bringing the hospital home: Ethical and social implications of high-tech care.* Baltimore, MD: Johns Hopkins University Press.

Benjamin, A. E., Matthias, R. E., Franke, T., Mills, L., Hasenfeld, Y., Matras, L., Stoddard, S., & Kraus, L. (1998). *Who's in charge? Who gets paid? A study of methods for organizing supportive services at home.* Los Angeles: University of California at Los Angeles.

Capitman, J., Abrahams, R., & Ritter, G. (1997). Measuring the adequacy of home care for frail elders. *Gerontologist, 37,* 303–313.

Carcagno, G. J., & Kemper, P. (1988). The evaluation of the national long term

care demonstration: An overview of the channeling demonstration and its evaluation. *Health Services Research, 23,* 1–22.
Degenholtz, H., Kane, R. A., & Kivnick, H. Q. (1997). Care-related preferences and values of elderly community-based LTC consumers: Can case managers learn what's important to clients? *Gerontologist, 37,* 767–776.
Eisler, P. (1996, November 11–12). Buyer beware: The hidden risks of home health care. *USA Today,* pp. 11B, 12B, and 13B (November 11) 1A and 2A (November 12).
Geron, S. M. (1997). *The home care satisfaction measures (HCSM): Study design and initial results of item analyses.* Boston: Boston University School of Social Work.
Geron, S. M., & Kane, R. A. (1991). *Design issues and requirements analysis for a quality assurance system for personal care aide (PCA) services in South Carolina.* Minneapolis: Long-Term Care DECISIONS Resource Center, University of Minnesota School of Public Health.
Harris-Wheling, J., Feasley, J. C., & Estes, C. L. (Eds.). (1995). *Real people, real problems: An evaluation of the Long-Term Care Ombudsman Programs of the Older Americans Act.* Washington, DC: Institute of Medicine.
Kane, R. A. (1988). The noblest experiment of them all: Learning from the national channeling evaluation. *Health Services Research, 23*(1), 189–198.
_____. (1995a). Expanding the home care concept: Blurring distinctions among home care, institutional care, and other long-term care services. *Milbank Quarterly, 73,* 161–186.
_____. (1995b). Decision-making, care plans, and life plans in long-term care: Can case managers take account of clients' values and preferences.? In L. B. McCullough & N. L. Wilson, (Eds.), *Long-term care decisions: Ethical and conceptual dimensions* (pp. 87–109). Baltimore, MD: Johns Hopkins University Press.
_____. (1999). Goals of home care: Therapeutic, compensatory, either, or both? *Journal of Aging and Health, 112,* 299–321.
Kane, R. A., & Caplan A. L. (Eds.). (1993). *Ethical conflict in the management of home care: The case manager's dilemma.* New York: Springer.
Kane, R. A., & Degenholtz, H. (1997a). Case management as a force for quality assurance and quality improvement in home care. *Journal of Aging and Social Policy, 9*(4), 5–28.
_____. (1997b). Assessing values and preferences: Should we, can we? *Generations, 21*(1), 19–24.
Kane, R. A., & Frytak, J. (1994). *Models for case management in long-term care: Interactions of case managers and home care providers* (report submitted to the U.S. Congress Office of Technology Assessment). Minneapolis: National LTC Resource Center, Institute for Health Services Research, School of Public Health, University of Minnesota.

Kane, R. A., Frytak, J., & Eustis, N. N. (1997). Agency approaches to common quality problems in home care. *Home Health Care Services Quarterly, 16*(1–2), 21–40.

Kane, R. A., Frytak, J., Thomas, C. K., & Eustis, N. N. (1995). *Best practices in home care quality assurance: Activities initiated by home care agencies.* Minneapolis: Institute for Health Services Research, School of Public Health, University of Minnesota.

Kane, R. A., Kane, R. L., Illston, L. H., & Eustis, N. N. (1994). Perspectives on home care quality. *Health Care Financing Review 16*(1), 69–90.

Kane, R. A., & Wilson, K. B. (1993). *Assisted living in the United States: A new paradigm for residential care of frail elderly people.* Washington, DC: American Association of Retired Persons.

Kane, R. L., Kane, R. A., Ladd, R. C., & Veazie, W. J. (1998). Variation in state spending for long-term care: Factors associated with a more balanced system. *Journal of Health Politics, Policy, and Law, 23*(2), 263–390.

Kinney, E. D, Freedman, J. A., & Loveland Cook, C. A. (1994). Quality improvement in community-based long-term care: Theory and reality. *American Journal of Law and Medicine, 20,* 59–77.

Ladd, R. C., Kane, R. L., Kane, R. A., & Neilsen, W. J. (1995). *State long-term care profiles* (report of the National LTC Mentoring Program). Minneapolis: Division of Health Services Research and Policy, University of Minnesota School of Public Health.

Mahoney, K. J., & Simon-Rusinowitz, L. (1997). Cash and counseling demonstration and evaluation: Start-up activities. *Journal of Case Management, 6*(1), 25–31.

Nerney, T., & Shumway, D. (1996). *Beyond managed care: Self-Determination for people with disabilities.* Concord: Institute on Disability, University of New Hampshire.

Shaughnessy, P. W., Crisler, K. S., Schlenker, R. E., Arnold, A., Kramer, A. M., Powell, M. S., & Hittle, D. F. (1994). Measuring and assuring the quality of home care. *Health Care Financing Review, 16*(1), 35–68.

Shaughnessy, P. W., Schlenker, R. E., & Hittle, D. F. (1994). Home health care outcomes under capitated and fee-for-service payment. *Health Care Financing Review, 16*(1), 187–222.

Susik, D. H. (1995). *Hiring home caregivers: The family guide to in-home eldercare.* San Luis Opispo, CA: American Source Books.

The Management Group. (1995). *Care management quality project assessment guide, revised July 14, 1995.* Madison, WI: Author (Available from The Management Group, 217 S. Hamilton Street, Suite 200, Madison, WI 53703.)

U.S. General Accounting Office. (1995). *Medicare allegations against ABC*

Home Health Care (GAO-OSI-95-17). Washington, DC: Government Printing Office.

———. (1997). *Medicare home health agencies certification process is ineffective in excluding problem agencies* (testimony before the Special Committee on Aging, U.S. Senate, GAO/T-HEHS-97-180). Washington, DC: U.S. Government Printing Office.

———. (1998). *Medicare Improper Activities by Mid-Delta Home Health.* (GAO/OSI-98-5). Washington, DC: U.S. Government Printing Office.

Weissert, W. G. (1988). The National Channeling Demonstration: What we knew, know now, and still need to know. *Health Services Research, 23*(1), 175–187.

Wiener, J. M., & Harris, K. M. (1990). Myths and realities: Why what most of what everybody knows about long-term care is wrong. *Brookings Review, 8*(4), 29–34.

Young, H. M., & Sikma, S. K. (1998). *The evaluation of the implementation of nurse delegation in Washington State.* Seattle: University of Washington School of Nursing.

SECTION FOUR

THE ISSUES AND CHALLENGES AHEAD

CHAPTER 11

The Uncertain Future of Home Care

Carroll L. Estes

Health care has been dramatically restructured as a result of more than a decade of health policy changes and cost containment efforts. Home care has experienced some of the most profound changes among all major players in the health industry. These changes are tantamount to a metamorphosis in which major transformations have occurred in the nature of services delivered, the clients served, the staffing patterns, and the organizational structures that provide these services.

Demand for home care services has risen with the restructuring of the health care delivery system, technological advances, and cost containment pressures that have pushed hospital lengths of stay to new lows while enabling an increasing array of procedures to be performed on an outpatient basis and in the home. Demographic trends will continue to augment the need for home care. The population age 65 and older grew 22% in the 1980s, more than double the growth of the nation's population, and it will at least double in the next 40 years. Those 85 and older, the fastest growing age group in America, are projected to increase nearly fivefold (from 4 million to 18 million) between 2000 and 2050, according to the middle series projections of the U.S. Bureau of the Census; the high series projections are almost twice that (U.S. Bureau of the Census, 1996a, 1996b). Even these startling figures could be an underestimate, as mortality rates have declined between 1970 and 1993 for older adults (Manton, Stallard, & Liu, 1993), especially among men (Kinsella, 1998). Manton and his colleagues report mortality declines of 8.6% for those 85 and older between 1988 and 1991 alone. By 2050, according to the middle series projections of the census, nearly one fourth of the population (78 million Americans) will be 65 and older, while total expenditures for nursing home care are projected to more than triple by 2030 (Friedland & Summer, 1999, p. 53).

There is new appreciation of the potential impact on home care of the baby boom, a cohort of 76 million Americans born between 1946 and 1964. The oldest members of this cohort turned age 50 in 1996 and by 2020 will be approaching age 70. Major fiscal problems for government programs, and especially Medicaid in terms of long-term care expenditures, are projected to occur around 2030, when the oldest boomers are "old old," age 85 and older (Congressional Budget Office, 1998a). Given that the elderly population will almost double in the next 50 years, the aging of the baby boom will create significant demand for and on home care services throughout the first half of the 21st century and beyond (U.S. General Accounting Office, 1998). The sheer volume of the number of elders is expected to augment the need for all kinds of long-term care services, despite the recent and projected reductions in rates of disability among the elderly (Rice, 1996). However, some have argued that a large and sustained increase in federally funded scientific research in biology and genetics will lessen the need for long-term care as well as other forms of care (Pardes et al., 1999).

HOME CARE UTILIZATION AND EXPENDITURES

The import of home care within the larger health care industry is illustrated by the fact that it has been the fastest growing segment of health care in the United States. In the mid-1990s, home care was the second fastest growing part of the U.S. economy as a whole. Between 1991 and 1993 Medicare home health care and nursing home care charted by far the two highest average annual percentage growth rates (37.7% and 46.4%, respectively). Both of these services were among the highest rates of expenditure growth for the 1984 to 1991 period as well—15.3% and 26.2%, respectively (Davis & Burner, 1995)—generating serious concern over the growth of these services and costs (Bishop & Skwara, 1993; Kenney & Moon, 1997).

By 1995 home care expenditures reached $26.6 billion, of which $14.3 billion was under Medicare and $4.3 billion was under Medicaid. In that same year, out of pocket expenditures of $5.5 billion for home care exceeded those of Medicaid, while private insurance paid a negligible proportion—about $300 million, or less than 1% (U.S. General Accounting Office, 1998; see also Burner & Waldo, 1995). Also in 1995, Medicare spent almost twice as much on home health care, $14.3 billion, as it did on nursing home care (U.S. General Accounting Office, 1998). Between 1990 and 1996 Medicare home health care expenditures rose from $3.9 billion to $18.3 billion (Moon, Gage, & Evans, 1997). Now, following the Balanced Budget Act of 1997 (BBA97), projections for Medicare home health expenditures in 2000 are at $19.0 billion (Congressional Budget Office, 1998b). Out-of-pocket costs of long-term care are a major financial burden on and of great concern to older persons and their families, who pay for 40% of these costs. Nevertheless, the federal government also plays a substantial role, accounting for about 45% of all spending in 1995 for nursing home and home care for the elderly (Congressional Budget Office, 1998a; U.S. General Accounting Office, 1998). Medicare funds one fourth and Medicaid funds one third of all long-term care expenditures, about 70% of which is for nursing home care (U.S. General Accounting Office, 1998). The fact that Medicare, Medicaid, and other public sources together pay for the lion's share of home care ($20.8 billion of the total of $26.6 billion in 1995) signifies the import of government policy and politics in determining the fate of the industry and those whom it serves.

According to the Congressional Budget Office's *Economic and Budget Outlook: 1999 to 2008,* although growth in payments for home health services (HHS) and skilled nursing facilities (SNFs) were the fastest growing areas of Medicare spending under fee-for-service (FFS) during the past decade, they are expected to slow in the first decade of the new millennium (Congressional Budget Office, 1998b). Reductions in the rate of spending increases in home care, as in SNF care, are a result of major changes incorporated in BBA97. For home health care in particular, the BBA initiated reductions in agency specific limits and limits related to per-enrollee spending that have slowed the growth of Medicare spending for home health care, the largest impact of which occurs in 2000 (Congressional Budget Office, 1998b). With the passage of BBA97, Medicare expenditure growth reductions were projected to be reduced by $115 billion between 1998 and 2002. The impact and implications of this legislation (Lewin Group, 1998) are discussed later in this chapter.

On the other hand, the *1998–1999 Occupational Outlook Handbook* of the Bureau of Labor Statistics reports that, between 1996 and 2000, the largest percentage of job growth—with the exception of computer and systems analysts (growing at 103% and 118%, respectively)—is projected for jobs related to home care. Employment change projections are for an increase of 85% for personal and home care aides and 76% for home health aides (Bureau of Labor Statistics, 1998). Four of the top 10 industries with the fastest job growth in the 1996–2000 period are health services (at 68%), residential care (at 59%), social services (at 50%), and health practitioners (at 47%) (Bureau of Labor Statistics, 1998).

Although there is still limited research on the effects of managed care on home care, research by Shaughnessy and his colleagues found that during a 19-month period the frequency of home care visits seemed to be constrained under HMOs—57 visits under FFS as compared 10 to 15 visits under HMOs (Schlenker et al., 1995; Shaughnessy et al., 1994a, 1994b). This same research also showed more adverse home health care outcomes for patients in managed care than in FFS settings (Schlenker, Shaughnessy, & Little, 1995; Shaughnessy, Schlenker, & Hittle, 1994a, 1994b). Ware, Bayliss, Rogers, Kosinski, and Tarlov (1996) has shown that the elderly and poor fare worse under HMOs than FFS. Similarly, social HMOs (S/HMOs), which integrate long-term care and acute care, do not seem effective with respect to long-term care services. An evaluation of S/HMOs conducted for the Health Care Financing Administration (HCFA) found that older persons who were impaired, or who were acutely ill and had chronic impairments, fared worse than the control group in FFS (Manton et al., 1993). These studies raise important questions about the quality and outcomes of care for the growing old-old population under managed care, which has a high incidence of chronic illness.

There is a lack of consensus about the appropriate use of home care, as suggested by the fact that home care utilization varies geographically (Schore, 1994; Welch, Wennberg, & Welch, 1996). Another question concerns the extent to which rising home care services and costs are attributable to or substituting for changes in hospital care (e.g., prospective payment system/PPS and reduced lengths of stay/LOS) and/or to other factors. Estes and her colleagues (Estes, Swan, & associates 1993), in research conducted between 1985 and 1988 on certified home health agencies regarding the effects of hospital PPS, concluded that these and other community-based services were profoundly affected as many older persons were discharged to home health care with shorter hospital LOS (Neu & Harrison, 1988; Spohn, Bergthold, & Estes, 1987–1988; Torrez, Estes, & Linkins, 1998; Wood & Estes, 1990). Based on later data, Welch and colleagues (1996) contend that Medicare home health care services do not replace hospital services, finding that 1993 population-based home health care utilization rates did not vary with lower hospital admission rates or shorter length of stay to predict service substitution. The difference in the findings of these two studies are likely due to the different roles played by home health care providers under Medicare immediately following the implementation of PPS (mid-1980s), compared to its role now, nearly a decade later. That Medicare home health care did serve a transitional function for earlier hospital discharges has been demonstrated for selected diagnosis-related groups (DRGs) (Kenney, 1991).

Bishop and Skwara (1993) and Welch and colleagues (1996) report that increases in Medicare home health care visits reflect the program's move toward providing long-term care (defined by Welch and associates as enrollee visits lasting 6 months or more). Lawsuits in the 1980s are credited for these changes in utilization. The 1997 BBA has stimulated further controversy about access to care and home health service utilization, as evidenced by a new round of legal actions including a lawsuit (*Healey vs. Shalala*) against HCFA (National Association for Home Care, 1998a; National Senior Citizens Law Center, 1998).

PERSPECTIVES ON THE TRANSFORMATION OF HOME CARE

The future of home care must be considered in the context of this dynamic and fluid environment and the major changes and demands that are projected for it. Work at the Institute for Health & Aging, University of California, San Francisco, and elsewhere, has demonstrated that home care is one of the most rapidly changing elements of the delivery system (Estes, Swan, & Associates, 1993).

Waves of Change in Home Care

Five major waves of change in home care have been identified in response to fiscal and policy changes from the 1980s to the present. Commencing with the budget cuts and block grants in the early 1980s under the Reagan administration, the *first wave* of change was the period of cutback management (1978–1981) following taxpayer revolts (such as California's Proposition 13) and the federal budget cuts in the 1981 Omnibus Budget Reconciliation Act (OBRA81). In home care, largely nonprofit and public home care agencies (e.g., Visiting Nurse Associations) sought to preserve their existing organizational infrastructures intact, as many sustained across the board cuts.

The *second wave* (1982–1983) of change was one of reorganization for efficiency in which home care providers began to respond to growing competition resulting from the encouragement of for-profit home care contained in the Omnibus Reconciliation Act of 1980 and subsequent Reagan administration cost containment and deregulatory policies. Market rhetoric grew as charges surfaced concerning the inefficiencies of nonprofit management and the "unfair competition" of nonprofits with proprietaries in health care (Estes, Binney, & Bergthold, 1989).

The *third wave* of change, extending from 1983 to the present, is one of full-fledged and increasingly intense competition and market restructuring. A combination of political and market forces and federal policy changes have promoted a blizzard of mergers and reorganizations, vertical and horizontal integration, and the growing dominance of proprietary providers of home care in a field that historically was public and nonprofit in character, also raising questions of access and the blurring of the boundaries between nonprofit and for-profit providers (Clarke & Estes, 1992; Estes & Swan, 1994; Estes et al., 1992). The *fourth wave* of change (which began in 1990) is one of managed care and system consolidation as home care and all other health providers attempt to survive by maintaining or expanding market share in a dynamic and rapidly changing environment.

The *fifth* wave of change is one of continuing fiscal pressure on government funding for home health care as reflected in BBA97. This legislation made the most significant changes to the Medicare program since the initiation of the prospective payment system for hospitals in

1983—and some say, since the enactment of Medicare itself in 1965 (Hafkenshiel, 1997; National Association for Home Care, 1998a, 1998b, 1988c). While the BBA extends the life of the program's funding, it produces higher premiums, reduced coverage, increased copayments and lowered capitation payments for HMOs, all of which are expected to affect older patients, particularly those who are vulnerable and living on the margins or in need of long-term care (Moon et al., 1997).

The restructuring of home care is reflected in a series of larger processes of change that have occurred in home-and community-based care during the past decade. Estes and colleagues (Estes, 1986; Estes et al., 1993) have identified a series of major transformative processes of community-based long-term care covering the period from 1983 to 1990 (Estes & Binney, 1997; Estes et al., 1993), all of which have touched home care in one way or another. The transformation of home care, appropriately described as the "metamorphosis of home care" (Humphers, Estes, & Bergthold, 1993), is reflected in the nine processes listed below:

- *Privatization* (the decline of public and nonprofit provision and growth of for-profits)
- *Fragmentation and unbundling of services* (the selling of single services that are more billable and profitable, and the decline of comprehensive service packages)
- *Competition* (increasing contest between for-profit and nonprofit providers vying for referrals, market share, and profits)
- *Rationalization of care provision* (vertical and horizontal integration across services and industries; the development of hybrid tax status entities; increased organizational size and complexity)
- *Informalization* (the transfer of services from the formal service sector to the informal sector of the home and community, mainly to women)
- *Medicalization of home- and community-based long-term care* (CBLTC) due to reimbursement schemes (e.g., Medicare and Medicaid) that reimburse for medical and skilled nursing/home health but not social supportive/nonmedical home care services) (Wood & Estes, 1990)
- *Labor restructuring* (increases in contract and part-time labor with lower career opportunities and fewer benefits for home care workers)
- *Stratification of care* (targeting clients who can pay privately vs. others)

- *Delegitimation of nonprofit service providers* (attacks on nonprofit service providers as inefficient and unfairly competitive with for-profit providers)

HOME CARE AND CONTEMPORARY POLICY CHANGES

The future of home care will be affected by a number of factors (Estes & Binney, 1997). Medicare cost cutting, through BBA97 and changing market forces, are likely to continue to impose relentless pressures to reduce expenditures for services in the home, to decrease home health visits, and to decrease home health revenues per visit. Marilyn Moon (1998) has projected that BBA provisions will lower Medicare home health care spending by $16.2 billion, or 12.8%, over a 5-year period. In order to limit the volume of services, patient eligibility and control costs, the BBA made numerous changes to Medicare's home health policy. These include prospective payment for home health care under Medicare (which will decrease or eliminate cost-based reimbursement for overhead) through cost caps per episode; the bundling of all post acute services—including rehabilitation, nursing home, and home care—into a single payment to hospitals, which, in turn, negotiate the lowest possible prices for postacute service providers; and caps on each 120 day episode of care, in addition to narrower criteria for determining the need for skilled nursing care.

Managed Care and the "Free Rider" Problem

The growth of managed care and HMOs, in itself, also will increase utilization control over home care and decrease industry self-regulation. The power shifts to insurers and the managed care industry from government and the FFS system are consequential for the services that come under the managed care umbrella, including home care (Rappaport, 1997). Postacute, subacute, and acute care services will continue to move from the hospital to the home. Medicaid cuts, welfare reform, and increased state discretion and power will exert downward pressures on the utilization of home-and community-based services paid for from public sources (e.g., Medicaid waiver packages). These and other forces (e.g., welfare reform and block grants), which have increased state discretion and reduced or eliminated national standards for eligibility and other benefit determinations, will increase problems of access to home care for those not able to purchase these services privately out of pocket. Home care will continue to be dramatically affected by the climate of crisis and cutbacks. The failure of the Bipartisan Commission on the Future of Medicare in 1999 to reach any consensus or plan to address the long-run solvency of Medicare, coupled with demographic population aging, means that the current cost pressures will only increase over the near term.

The rapid growth of managed care and federal policy to stimulate more use of it by Medicare enrollees raises questions concerning home care for older persons (Feder & Moon, 1998). Among the most salient with regard to elderly and disabled people are whether home care will be more or less accessible under managed care, how access to home care will be affected, and with what consequences, for those needing long-term care, and what the health outcomes, cost, and quality of home care will be under managed care compared to FFS or other alternatives.

The free rider problem has been described by Uwe Reinhart as a situation in which people "ride" or "mooch" on the system (Reinhart, 1995) without fully paying their way (or paying nothing). The potential "free rider problem" in home care (Estes & Linkins, 1997) concerns what new "uses" (or support) will managed care organizations extract from home-and community-based care in their drive to further reduce costly lengths of stay in hospitals, ambulatory care, and day surgeries. How many resources of the social supportive services in the community and increases in the informal (family and friends) care work will be required in the drive of managed care organizations to better the bottom line? What will be the transfer (if any) of "saved" resources and profits of managed care to compensate or pay for the increased CBLTC services that are (and will be) drawn upon in order to achieve the cost savings of individual managed care corporations?

The situation may be appropriately described using O'Connor's (1973) concept of the socialization of the costs of capital in which managed care corporations mooch off of an increasingly stressed community delivery system that is a public resource, largely funded by public monies and operated through the nonprofit sector agencies, with the simultaneous privatization of the profits of capital, as managed care companies make profits extracted from their operations and from the public and the community. There are public and private costs that managed care entities pass on to the public in their decisions to reduce costs and increase profits (e.g., practices such as "drive by" or "drive through" deliveries, "dumping" of patients who may then require considerable supportive services, and family and community work not paid for by managed care entities). The costs to patients, the community, and the public are likely to be significant, yet these costs are largely and routinely uncalculated in the outcome methodologies that are incorporated in current measurement approaches. First, the outcome measures are calculated for patients in individual plans and corporations; they do not account for the costs that are shifted "out of plan" onto the individual patients themselves, their families, and friends ("informal" costs) in terms of such consequences of lost days of work compensation, changes in employment, and/or increased out-of-pocket expenses for caregiving of postoperative or chronically ill family members. The measurement systems also do not account for either the public health costs or the overall outcomes in terms of community health indicators, risk selection and risk-aversion patterns, and costs shifted to public and nonprofit institutions.

The Problem of the "No Care Zone"

The increased enrollment of elders in managed care and its effects on home care now come after more than a decade of Medicare cost containment, including PPS that gives hospitals an incentive for the early discharge of older patients. With the introduction of the PPS and DRGs, 27 million days of hospital care were transferred to the home and community, which generated a "margin" (i.e., profit) for hospitals of approximately $3 billion in the first year alone (Estes, 1987). This occurred while there was virtually no transfer of the "costs" of the care burden from the hospital to support community-based services and informal caregivers that provided the work of caring for patients who began to be discharged earlier from the hospital. The increasing pressure on a variety of CBLTC providers by PPS, in a climate of constrained and declining social service funding, produced a "no care zone" (Estes et al., 1993), in which elders who need services or social supports either intermittently or continuously are unable to obtain them unless they are able to privately assemble and pay for them.

Today the question is whether, with the incentives of managed care to cut costs wherever possible, a similar process is occurring of "dumping" and "bumping down" of older persons and patients out of managed care settings and onto the CBLTC system and women and families. Also at issue is how implementation of the 1997 BBA prospective payment for home health care, and other changes imposed on HMOs as well, will affect the incentive systems to utilize (or avoid or minimize) home care services and whether the services and costs of HMOs, more generally, expand Medicare enrollment in managed care plans as much as projected. A related question concerns whether the changes under managed care will create their own social iatrogenic effects through the production of increased forms of dependency among patients and, more broadly, in the population (Estes, 1993). The previously cited recent research on the poorer outcomes of HMOs compared to FFS for home care (Shaughnessey et al. 1994a, 1994b) and by Ware and colleagues (1996) showing that older and disabled patients experience better outcomes in FFS than in managed care. intensify the import of this question: Will the no care zone grow under managed care?

POLITICAL AND ECONOMIC CHALLENGES TO HOME CARE

The challenge to home care and the future of long-term care will be a product of multiple factors:

- the sociodemographics of population aging and the younger disabled population
- greater awareness of home care services and activism by home care patients and their families
- technological advances enabling more ambulatory care and services to be provided in the home
- judicial rulings expanding home care services eligibility
- increased managed care
- shortened hospital stays
- a decline in nursing home use
- the strong preference of elders for services in the home and community rather than institutions

In addition, there will be other political and economic factors.

Political Factors

The power of corporations, particularly insurance and managed care corporations, has dramatically enhanced their ability to shape, if not direct, the policy agenda in ways that create change and uncertainty for the home care industry and its patients. Resource and regulatory struggles between the nursing home and home care industries are expected to intensify since the states have augmented discretion to alter their funding commitments under welfare reform and the block grants for social, mental health, and other services, as well as strong political pressures to contain Medicaid costs. A fragmented unorganized series of home-and community-care agencies are pitted against the traditionally more influential nursing home and managed care interests in struggles to preserve and expand their traditional state and other funding bases. Similar struggles are being played out many times over in the different states between insurers, managed care companies, and home care and other service providers in the long-term care continuum. Further affecting the resources available and the direction of home care are the outcomes of highly charged partisan struggles in Congress and with the White House concerning the fate of Medicare and Medicaid and the decisions of the governors and state legislatures intent on tax reductions and cost containment despite the fact that many states are enjoying rather significant state surpluses in the late 1990s. The present tensions over the implementation of BBA97 are but one example.

Economic Factors

The rising for-profit concentration in all aspects of the medical industrial complex have vastly increased the stakes in the profitability of health and home care (Estes, Harrington, & Pellow, 2000). A contradiction is that rising health costs may signify healthier profit margins, while at the same time generating oppositional forces to the rising costs from the segments of the public and private sectors that must pay for them. In the U.S. economic system, the costs of business profitability in health are "socialized," in that they are subsidized by government funding for medical care, tax subsidies for health insurance, and a public sector that pays for fully 40% of the health care dollars spent. The public sector does not compete as a service provider with the for-profit sector. Rather, it serves primarily as provider of last resort. At the same time, the profits of the trillion-dollar medical industrial complex are privatized; they are not turned back to the public sector.

The larger political and economic context is one in which health care restructuring is driven by the private sector through market forces rather than a national health policy of universal insurance. The context is also one in which there is uncertainty regarding the fate of long-term care, as it remains largely (and increasingly) the purview of the states in the absence of federal policy on long-term care. Recent changes in Medicare under BBA97 have intensified uncertainty for the home care industry and for those who require care in the home (Lewin Group, 1998). The Congressional Budget Office estimated that the BBA97 changes would save $16 billion through 2002, in large part by changing the reimbursement of home health from a cost basis (subject to limits) to a per-beneficiary cost limit, followed by a prospective payment system in 1999. By late 1998 the interim payment system (IPS) had reduced per-visit cost limits an average of 21%. One analysis estimated that reimbursement would decline by 30% in fiscal year 1998, and Medicare home health expenditures would have declined from a projected $20 billion to $17.8 billion, also in 1998 (National Association for Home Care, 1998d).

A study by the Lewin Group (1998) identified a number of problems for home health providers stemming from the implementation of BBA97. The per-beneficiary limits in BBA97, for example, may create financial disincentives for agencies to care for patients with more intensive care needs. Advances in the work on case mix adjustment and prospective payment methodologies are required, and their implementation is fraught with potentially serious issues for patients, for the industry, and for the role of home care in the long term care system of services. The types of agencies most affected by BBA97, according to the Lewin report (1998), include those with increased severity in their case mix since 1994, small agencies with a large percentage of high use and rural agencies where alternative sources of care are unavailable, and agencies created through mergers and acquisitions. One concern is the number of home health agency closures between 1997 and 1998. The National Association for Home Care (1998e) reports that 760 such agencies closed nationwide, while a survey of state health departments by the National Association for Home Care (Lewin Group, 1998) reports a significantly higher number. These closures followed the period 1996–1997 when the growth rate of home care decelerated from a projected 13.8% to 4.8% (National Association for Home Care Agencies, 1998f). Strategies that home health agencies may pursue to remain under the BBA97–imposed cost limits (e.g., reducing frequency of visits or level of staff) could negatively affect not only the industry but also Medicare beneficiaries in need of services. The denial of services, in turn, could both increase the patient's risk of institutionalization and caregiver strain.

Particularly vulnerable are those who need nonmedical home care services, such as chronically ill older persons and those younger severely disabled adults with high-intensity needs requiring care of long duration and who have obtained in-home supportive assistance from a home health aide while also getting skilled home care. Patient advocates are increasingly vocal about their concerns, with political and legal actions and the mobilization of coalitions of the younger disabled and the elderly to challenge federal and state policy on numerous fronts. Two national class action lawsuits were filed in 1998. In one, Medicare home health beneficiaries with severe disabilities joined the National Spinal Cord Injury Association in a national class action lawsuit against HCFA, challenging the "confined to home" requirement used to deny otherwise qualified patients coverage for critically needed home care services (National Association for Home Care, 1998a). The National Association for Home Care is also preparing a lawsuit against the HCFA concerning low per-beneficiary limits (National Association for Home Care, 1998b). Another lawsuit by Medicare home health patients in Connecticut, Alabama, Massachusetts, Michigan, and New Jersey charges the Secretary of the U.S. Department of Health and Human Services with failure to require Medicare-certified home health agencies to provide basic due process rights to patients before denying or terminating services to them (National Senior Citizens Law Center, 1998). These are consumer responses to a new wave of HCFA denials of claims for home health patients, stemming from the financial squeeze on home health agencies because of the implementation of BBA97.

THE FUTURE OF HOME CARE: MAJOR QUESTIONS

Central questions revolve around the fate of Medicare and Medicaid, as well as long-term care policy more broadly. In all three of these policy arenas, what will be the funding, eligibility, and regulations for both the medical and nonmedical services that are under the rubric of home care? Attacks on entitlement and the rhetoric of crisis and bankruptcy are being used to promote potentially drastic changes in these programs, with privatization, vouchers, benefit cuts, and for-profit managed care strongly competing with the more traditional fee-for-service system.

The future challenges to home care are profound. The larger goal of home care policy should be to embrace social as well as economic objectives in offering home care that is accessible, affordable, and universal.

This necessitates an approach that contains three elements. Future policies should (1) empower consumers rather than generate dependency; (2) not exploit families, or the largely nonprofit social service system that is a core element of the safety net, or employed workers who are the safety net caregivers; and (3) reflect a socially just approach to home care recipients and home care workers (both informal and formal) by promoting gender, ethnic, intergenerational, and class justice.

REFERENCES

Axene, D. V., & Hulet, J. J. (1994, April). *The emerging role of managed home care.* Paper presented on behalf of Milliman & Roberson, Inc. at a meeting on Reengineering Home Care for Capitation, California Association for Health Services at Home, Sacramento, CA.

Bishop, C., & Skwara, K. C. (1993). Recent growth of Medicare home health. *Health Affairs, 12*(3): 95–110.

Bureau of Labor Statistics. (1998). *1998–1999 occupational outlook handbook.* PilotM@bls.gov/ooh.table2.htm.

Burner, S. T., & Waldo, D. R. (1995). National health expenditure projections, 1994–2005. *Health Care Financing Review, 16*(1), 221–242.

Clarke, L., & Estes, C. L. (1992). Sociological and economic theories of markets and nonprofits: Evidence from home health organizations. *American Journal of Sociology, 97*(4), 945–969.

Congressional Budget Office. (1998a). *Long term budgetary pressures and policy options.* Washington, DC: U.S. Government Printing Office.

———. (1998b). *Economic and budget outlook: Fiscal years 1999–2008.* Washington, DC: U.S. Government Printing Office.

Davis, M. H., & Burner, S. T. (1995). Three decades of Medicare: What the numbers tell us. *Health Affairs, 14*(4), 236–241.

Estes, C. L. (1986). The politics of ageing in America. *Ageing and Society, 6*(2), 121–134.

———. (1987). *Testimony on the President's FY 1988 budget proposals* (hearing before the U.S. House of Representatives Committee on Ways and Means, Subcommittee on Health). Washington, DC: Government Printing Office.

———. (1993). The aging enterprise revisited. *Gerontologist, 3,* 292–298.

Estes, C. L., & Binney, E. A. (1997). The restructuring of home care. In D. M. Fox & C. Raphael (Eds.), *Home based care for a new century* (pp. 5–21). New York: Milbank Memorial Fund and Blackwell Publishing.

———. (1989). The biomedicalization of aging: Dangers and dilemmas. *Gerontologist, 29,* 587–596.

Estes, C. L., Binney, E. A., & Bergthold, L. (1989). The role of ideology and public policy: The delegitimation of the nonprofit sector. In V. Hodgkinson & R. Lyman (Eds.), *The future of the nonprofit sector* (pp. 21–40). San Francisco: Jossey-Bass.

Estes, C. L., Harrington, C., & Pellow, D. (2000). The medical industrial complex. In E. Borgatta and M. Borgatta (Eds.), *The encyclopedia of sociology* (2nd ed., Vol. 3). New York: Macmillan.

Estes, C. L., & Linkins, K. W. (1997). Devolution and aging policy: Racing to the bottom in long term care? *International Journal of Health Service, 27*(3), 427–442.

Estes, C. L., & Swan, J. H. (1994). Privatization and access to home health care. *Milbank Quarterly, 72*(2), 277–298.

Estes, C. L., Swan, J. H., & associates. (Eds.). (1993). *The long term care crisis.* Newbury Park, CA: Sage.

Estes, C. L., Swan, J. H., Bergthold, L. A., & Hanes-Spohn, P. (1992). Running as fast as they can: Organizational changes in home health care. *Home Health Care Services Quarterly, 13*(1/2): 35–69.

Estes, C. L., & Wood, J. B. (1993). Waves of change. In C. L. Estes, J. H. Swan, & associates (Eds.), *The long term care crisis* (pp. 210–224). Newbury Park, CA: Sage.

Feder, J., & Moon, M. (1998). Managed care for the elderly: A threat or a promise? *Generations, 29*(2), 6–10.

Franklin, J. C. (1997, November). Industry output and employment projections to 2006. *Monthly Labor Review,* pp. 39–54.

Friedland, R. B., & Summer, L. (1999). *Demography is not destiny.* Washington, DC: National Academy on an Aging Society and the Gerontological Society of America.

Hafkenshiel, J. (1997). Home health reimbursement and the 1997 Budget Act. *Home Care Provider, 2*(6), 279–281.

Humphers, S., Estes, C. L., & Bergthold, L. (1993). The metamorphosis of home care. In C. L. Estes, J. H. Swan, & associates (1993), *The long term care crisis* (pp. 93–111). Newbury Park, CA: Sage.

Kenney, G. M. (1991). Understanding the effects of PPS on Medicare home health use. *Inquiry, 28*(2), 129–139.

Kenney, G. M., & Moon, M. (1997). *Reining in the growth in home health services under Medicare.* New York: The Commonwealth Fund.

Kinsella, K. G. (1998). *The trends that are important for business.* Washington, DC: U.S. Bureau of the Census.

Lewin Group. (1998). *Implications of the Medicare home health interim payment system of the 1997 Balanced Budget Act* (report prepared for the National Association of Home Care, March 13). Washington DC: The Lewin Group (www.nahc.org/NAHC/NewsInfo/98nr/lewinrpt.html).

Manton, K. G., Newcomer, R., Lowrimore, G. R., Vertrees, J. C., & Harrington, C. (1993). Social/health maintenance organization and fee-for-service health outcomes over time. *Health Care Financing Review* (2), 173–202.

Manton, K. G., Stallard, E., & Liu, K. (1993, September). Forecasts of active life expectancy: Policy and fiscal implications [Special issue]. *Journal of Gerontology, 48,* 11–26.

Moon, M., Gage, B., & Evans, A. (1997). *An examination of key Medicare provisions in the BBA of 1997.* New York: Commonwealth Fund.

National Association for Home Care. (1998a). *Medicare home health care patients file class action lawsuit against Health Care Financing Administration.* May 6 (www.nahc.org/NAHC/NewsInfo/98nr/lewinrpt.html).

———. (1998b). *NAHC prepares lawsuit against Health Care Financing Administration.* April 1. (www.nahc.org/NAHC/NewsInfo/98nr/lewinrpt.html).

———. (1998c). *Study finds Medicare home health interim payment system may affect most vulnerable patients.* March 16 (www.nahc.org/NAHC/NewsInfo/98nr/lewinrpt.html).

———. (1998d). *Medicare home health care interim payment system is inherently unfair to patients and providers.* July 15 (www.nahc.org/NAHC/NewsInfo/98nr/lewinrpt.html).

———. (1998e). *Official state data reveal more than doubling of home health agency closures.* October 2 (www.nahc.org/NAHC/NewsInfo/98nr/lewinrpt.html).

National Center for Health Statistics. (1998). *Vital statistics of the U.S.: 1995* (Vol. 2, Part A, Section 6). Hyattsville, MD: U.S. Department of Health and Human Services.

National Senior Citizens Law Center. (1998). Medicare home health care patients sue to enforce due process rights when care is terminated or reduced. *NSCLC Washington Weekly, 24*(11), 41, & 43.

Neu, C. R. & Harrison, S. C. (1988). *Posthospital care before and after the Medicare prospective payment system.* Santa Monica, CA: RAND.

Newcomer, R. J., Harrington., C., & Kane, R. L. (Eds.). (1996). Managed care in acute and primary care settings. In R. Newcomer & A. Wilkinson (Eds.), *Annual review of gerontology and geriatrics* (Vol. 16, pp. 1–36). New York: Springer.

O'Connor, J. (1973). *Fiscal crisis of the state.* New York: St. Martin's Press.

Pardes, H., Manton, K. G., Lander, E. S., Tolley, H. D., Ullian, A. D., & Palmer, H. (1999). Effects of medical research on health care and the economy. *Science, 283,* 36–37.

Rappaport, M. (1997). *Home health care in the context of managed care.* Ph.D. doctoral dissertation. San Francisco: University of California, San Francisco.

Reinhardt, U. (1995). Health reform is dead! Long live health reform! *Trends in Health Care, Law and Ethics, 10*(1/2), 7–10, 32.

Rice, D. P. (1996). Medicare beneficiary profile: Yesterday, today and tomorrow. *Health Care Financing Review, 18*(18), 23–46.

Schlenker, R. E., Shaughnessy, P. W., & Hittle, D. F. (1995). Patient-level cost of home care under capitated & fee-for-service payment. *Inquiry, 32,* 252–270.

Schore, J. R. (1994). *Patient, agency and area characteristics associated with regional variation in the use of Medicare home health services.* Princeton, NJ: Mathematica Policy Research.

Schore, J., Brown, R., & Phillips, B. (1993). *Medicare home health episodes, 1990/1991: Distributions of episode length and number of visits provided per episode* (report submitted to Health Care Financing Administration). Princeton, NJ: Mathematica Policy Research.

Shaughnessy, P. W., Schlenker, R. E., Hittle, D. F., & associates (1994a). *A study of home health care quality and cost under capitated and fee-for-service payment systems* (Vol. 1). Denver: University of Colorado, Center for Health Policy Research.

———. (1994b). Home health care outcomes under capitated and fee-for-service payment. *Health Care Financing Review, 16*(1), 187–222.

Spohn, P. H., Bergthold, L., & Estes, C. L. (1987–1988). From cottages to condos: The expansion of the home care industry under Medicare. *Home Health Care Services Quarterly, 8*(4), 25–55.

Torrez, D., Estes, C. L., & Linkins, K. (1998). The impact of a decade of policy on home health care utilization. *Home Health Care Services Quarterly, 16*(4), 35–6.

U.S. Bureau of the Census. (1996a). *Population projections of the U.S. by age, race, sex and Hispanic origin: 1995–2050.* Washington, DC: U.S. Government Printing Office.

———. (1996b). *65+ in the United States.* Washington, DC: U.S. Government Printing Office.

———. (1998). *Long term care: Baby boom generation presents financing challenges* (testimony of W. J. Scanlon, March 9, GAO/T-HEHS-98-107). Washington, DC: U.S. Government Printing Office.

Ware, J. E., Bayliss, M. S., Rogers, W. H., Kosinski, M., & Tarlov, A. R. (1996). Differences in 4-year health outcomes for elderly and poor, chronically ill patients treated in HMO and fee-for-service systems. *Journal of the American Medical Association, 276,* 1039–1047.

Welch, G. H., Wennberg, D. E., & Welch, W. P. (1996). The use of Medicare home health services. *New England Journal of medicine, 335,* 324–329.

Wood, J. B., & Estes, C. L. (1990). The impact of DRGs on community-based service providers: Implications for the elderly. *American Journal of Public Health, 80,* 840–843.

INDEX

('i' indicates an illustration; 't' indicates a table)

Accountability, home health care, 222–223
Accreditation
 home health agencies, 216
 JCAHO, 124
Action plans
 OBQI, 176–177
 QA, 220–221
Activities of daily living (ADLs), 6, 37, 83
Activity-based cost accounting, home health care agencies, 128
Adult daughters, as home care workers, 87
Adult foster care, 47
Advance directives, 70
Adverse consequences, home health care, 71
Advocacy, 231
African Americans, communication style, 86
Agency-level predictors, resource consumption, 148, 150–152
Aging population. *See* Elderly
Alzheimer's disease, care costs, 15
American Association of Homes and Services for Aging, 12
American Association of Homes for the Aging, 12
American Medical Association, physician home health care guidelines, 201

Andersen behavioral model, resource consumption, 149
Asian Americans, communication style, 86, 87
Asset sheltering, 17
Assisted living facilities (ALFs), 47, 211
Asymmetrical family-worker relationship, 93–94

Baby boom cohort, 18, 19–20, 27
Balanced Budget Act of 1997 (BBA97), xiii, 24, 25, 241–242, 243, 244–245, 246
 IPS, 143, 155, 191
 problems resulting from, 251–252
Batch-level expenses, activity-based cost accounting, 128
Bereavement care, hospice service, 106
"Blended families," 20
"Brink of death" care, 108
Broker role, of family in home care, 81, 90–91
Business-level expenses, activity-based cost accounting, 129

Cancer, and hospice care, 109, 109t
Cardiac home care, 61–62
"Care for life," 16
Caregiving, 13–14. *See also* Family caregivers
Care stratification, home health care, 245

257

Case examples, home care assessment, 226
Case management, long-term care, 51
Case managers, QA role, 218, 229
Channeling Demonstration, 7. *See also* National Long Term Care Demonstration
Chronic illness, and home care, 44, 45
Chronic obstructive pulmonary disease (COPD), TM/HBHC study, 199
Civilian Health and Medical Program of the Uniformed Services (CHAMPUS), 105
Client, care recipient, 80
Clinical health status, resource consumption, 153, 154
Cognitively impaired, family roles in home care, 83
Collegial family-worker relationship, 94
Communication styles, in home care, 86–87
Community-based care, evaluation of, 194
Comorbidity, 36–37
Companion/sitter, 119
Compensatory goals, home health care, 223–224
Competition, home health care, 245
Complaint resolution, 231
Comprehensive Health Evaluation and Social Support project (CHESS), 64
Computer-assisted quality assurance (QA), 224–225
ComputerLink project, 63–64
Computer technology, and home care, 65
Condition-specific home team, high risk patients, 192–193
Congestive heart failure (CHF)
 NMHHC study, 201, 202–203
 TM/HBHC study, 199
Congressional Budget Office, estimates of future long-term care, 19
Connecticut Hospice, New Haven, 103

Consumer-oriented approach, QA, 215, 217, 229
Contextual factors, family home care, 86–87
Continuing care retirement communities (CCRCs), 16
Continuous care, 119
Continuous quality improvement (CQI)
 OBQI, 175–176
 QA, 213–214
Continuum of health care, home care in, 22
Contractual agencies, outcomes, 166–167, 167i
Control, and family caregiving, 91
Coordination, formal/informal caregiving, 13, 14
Cost containment, long-term care, 95
Cost-effectiveness, home health care services, 120–121, 130
"Cost-of-quality curve," home care, 25
Costs
 home care technology, 69
 HBPC study, 196, 197
 long-term care, 14–15
 OBQI, 181–182, 182i, 183, 186
Crisis management, hospice care, 108
Critical pathway development, home health care agencies, 130–131
Culture, and family in home care, 86
Current Population Survey (CPS) of 1987–89, home health care aides, 84
Custodial care, 47–48, 223
Customer satisfaction, home health care agencies, 126

Deductibility, long-term care insurance, 24
Deinstitutionalization, 209–210
Demand characteristics, family home care, 82–86
Dementia, family roles in home care, 83
Demonstration program, OBQI, 178
Demonstration projects, possible home health care, 229–232

Department of Veterans Affairs (DVA), health care system, 195
Diagnosis-related groups (DRGs), requiring home care, 5
Disability in old age, future increases in, 18, 19
Disability rates, decline in, 37
Discharge disposition, resource consumption, 153–154
Discharge, OBQI, 172, 173
Discharge planning, nurses involvement in, 66
Disease-state management programs, 120
Domiciliary care, 47
"Downsizings," home health care, 117
Dual-eligibles, 157, 231
Duggan v. Bowen (1988), 9
"Dumping" of patients, 247–248
Durable medical equipment, 119, 120i
Dying, at home, 69, 70

Educational approach, QA, 215, 218–219
Elderly
  demographic trends, 18–19, 35, 41, 42t, 239–240
  and disabled as allies, 27
  home care resource consumption, 139
Enabling factors, resource consumption, 149, 150, 213
End of life care, 101
End-stage management, hospice level, 107
Enterprise-level expenses, activity-based cost accounting, 129
Episode of care, unit of analysis, 146, 183
"Episode perspective," 145
Ethics, home care, 69–71
Ethnicity, and family in home care, 86
"Everyday families," 95

Family
  changing definition of, 95
  as proper context of care, 88, 89
  roles, in home care, 81, 82i, 87–94
Family caregivers, 13, 19–20
  aging of, 4
  cost relief, 26
  and high-tech home care, 67
  paid programs for, 88
  rights of, 95
  support of, 96
Federal Dependent Care Tax Credit, 95
Federal funding, long-term care, 23, 24
Fee-for-service (FFS)
  agencies, outcomes, 166–170, 167i, 168i, 169i
  patient outcomes, 157, 166, 242
Financial management, home health care agencies, 123
Formal family-worker relationship, 93
Formal home care, advantages of, 209
Formal sources of care, use of, 78–79
Fragmentation/unbundling, home health care, 245
"Free rider" problem, 247–248
Functional health status, resource consumption, 153, 154
Functional Independence Measure (FMI), rehabilitation, 174
Functional limitations, long-term home care, 6
Future trends
  demand for home care, 18–19
  family caregiving, 19–20

Geographic variation, home health care, 152, 242
Goal conflict, home health care, 224

Health care, long-term and home care as part of, 22, 28
Health Care Financing Administration (HCFA), 9
  home health care agencies, 131–132
  hospice funding, 104
  legal action against, 252
  OBQI Demonstration program, 178
  physician oversight, 22
  PPS, 138, 143, 144, 145–147, 155, 191–192, 243, 246
Health Insurance Manual (HFCFA's), 10

Index

Health Maintenance Organizations (HMOs), 124
  agencies, outcomes, 166–170, 167i, 168i, 169i
  patient outcome, 166, 242
  telephone-triage, 64
Health professionals
  challenges of home care, 21–23
  home care technology use, 65–66
Hemodialysis, at home, 63
High-risk patients, home care innovations, 192–193
High-tech home care, 46, 59, 84, 85, 195
Hispanics, communication style, 87
Home, definition, 39, 79
Home-and-community-based services (HCBS), funds for, 11, 26
Home Based Primary Care (HBPC), DVA, 195–197
Homebound, definition of, 140
Home care
  as alternative structure, 209–211
  belief in cost effectiveness, 8
  definition, 38–39
  four models of, 195
  innovations, 192–193
  Medicaid eligibility criteria, 141
  Medicare eligibility criteria, 140–142
  patient criteria, 213
  quality assurance in, 208, 227–232
Home care agencies, 120, 121
Home care ethics guidelines, 70
Home care industry
  growth of, 12, 40, 40t
  services of, 39
Home care physician, high risk patients, 192–193
Home care resource consumption, units of analysis, 142–148
Home Care Satisfaction Measures, 225
Home health agencies
  Medicare-certified, 138
  number of 40t
  QA, 220–221
  regulatory standards, 216, 222
Home health aides, 84, 147, 148

Home health care
  access to, 96–97
  baby boomer impact, 240
  economic factors of, 250–252
  expenditures for, 137–138, 163–164, 191–192, 241
  future challenges to, 249–252
  future policy for, 253
  goals of, 46
  growth, 117, 240–241. *See also* Medicare, Medicaid
  market segments, 120, 120i
  projected expenditures, 241–242
  recent changes in, 244–246
  research needs, 49–51
  resource consumption predictors, 148–153
  service fragmentation, 86
  sources of payment for, 43t
  state role, 221–222
  types of services used, 43t, 43–44
  users of, 41, 42t
Home health care teams, 132
Home health services
  growth reversal, 25
  reimbursement for, 4–5, 85
Homemaker service, 39, 48, 84
Home visit
  length of, 144–145
  staff mix, 147–148
  unit of analysis, 142–144
Hospice, 39
Hospice and Palliative Nurses Association, 112
Hospice care, 47, 102
  diagnoses, 108–109, 109t
  growth of, 105–106
  home care model, 195
  recipients, 109–110
  reimbursement, 9, 105, 107
  settings, 107–109
  TM/HBHC study, 199
Hospice house, 106
Hospice movement, 103, 104
Hospice team, 110–111
Hospitalization, need for, 243

Index

Household changes and aids, 61

Independence, valuation by older
  persons, 88
Informalization, home health care, 245
Informal sources of care, use of, 78
Information management, home health
  care agencies, 123, 131
Information technology, in home care,
  63–65, 72
Infusion sets, home use, 60
Infusion therapy, at home, 63, 84, 119,
  120i, 120
Institutional isomorphism, 151
Instrumental activities of daily living
  (IADLs), 6, 83
  Medicaid funds for, 11
Instrumental outcome, OBQI, 173
Insurance, long-term care, 15–16, 23, 24
Interim Payment system, Medicare, 143–
  144, 191
Intermittent care, 118
  definition of, 140, 143
Interpersonal dynamics, home care
  worker-client, 92

Job growth, home health industry, 242
Joint Commission on Accreditation of
  Health Care Organizations
  (JCAHO), 124

Katz Dependence Scale, 149
Kelly Assisted Living, 118
Kevorkian, Jack, 114
Kinship networks, changes in, 20
Kubler-Ross, Elizabeth, 114

Labor force, restructured home health
  care, 245
Legal issues, in home care, 69–71, 252
"Life care at home" (LCAH), 16
Living wills, 70
Long-term care (LTC)
  definition, 36
  expense of, 14, 15, 16
  as federal employee benefit, 27
  as health care, 28
  at home, 6
  maturation of, 35–36
  Medicare and Medicaid financing, 7
  policies, 95
  "Long-term Care Initiative," 25–26
Long-term care insurance, business of,
  24
Low-tech home care, 47, 48, 84, 85, 195

Managed care
  and home care, 25 246–249
  and home care business, 121–122,
    124–126, 125i
  home visit constraints, 242
  patient outcomes, 153, 156–157, 164,
    165–166, 242
Management Information System (MIS),
  possible demonstration project, 230
Marketing, home health care agencies,
  122
Market share, home health care agencies,
  126
Market/systemic approach, QA, 215,
  217–218
Means testing, 23
Mechanical ventilation, home use, 60,
  85, 119
Medicaid
  benefit coverage, 208
  estate planning, 17
  home care eligibility criteria, 141,
    157–158
  home health care expenditures, 138,
    153, 163–164, 241
  home health care growth, 5, 7, 11, 12,
    40, 41
Medical education, and home care, 22
Medical social worker, home visit, 148
Medical technologies, home use, 14, 59–60
Medicalization, home health care, 245
Medicare
  benefit coverage, 208
  home care benefits, 139
  home care eligibility criteria, 140–142,
    157–158

Medicare *(continued)*
  home health care expenditures, 137–138, 153, 163–164, 191–192, 240–241
  home health care growth, 5, 7, 9, 101, 12, 40, 41
  home health care obstacles, 203–204 IPS, 143–144, 191
  OBQI Demonstration program, HCFA, 178
  physician disincentives, 201
Medicare-certified home health care, 118–119
"Medicare-certified mindset," 129
Medicare Health Insurance Manual (HIM-11)
  homebound, 140
  intermittent, 143
  part-time, 143
Medicare Hospice Benefit (MHB), 104, 105, 108
  eligibility, 106–107
  informed consent, 110
Medicare/Medicaid, federal spending limitations, 23
Medicare skilled home care, 195
Medicare Survey and Certification Program, HCFA, 172
Minimum Data Set (MDS), nursing homes, 174
"Mobile health care delivery network," 132
Monitor role, of family in home care, 81, 91–92

Narcotics, in hospice care, 108–107, 113
National Association for Home Care (NAHC)
  agency closings, 251
  legal action against HCFA, 252
  survey, 124
National Board for Certification of Hospice and Palliative Nurses, 112
National Caregiver Support Program, 26
National Hospice Organization, 102

National Long Term Care Demonstration, 193–194
National Spinal Cord Injury Association, legal action against HCFA, 252
National Survey of Home and Hospital Care (1996), 40
Need factors, resource consumption, 149–150, 156
Negligence claims, 71
"No care zone," 248
Nonprofit providers, delegitimation of, 246
Normalization, caregiving responsibilities, 90
Northwest Memorial Home Health Care, Inc. (NMHHC) study, 201
Nurses
  and home care, 22, 120, 120i
  home care technology use, 65–66
  home visits, 147, 148
  in hospice care, 111–112
  litigation risks, 71
Nursing homes
  cost containment, 7
  expenditures for, 240–241

Occupational Outlook Handbook (1998–1999), home health industry, 242
Older American Act, 139
Oldest old population, 35
Omnibus Reconciliation Act of 1980 (ORA80), 8
Omnibus Budget Reconciliation Act of 1981 (ORA81), 11, 244
One-stop operation, home health care agencies, 121
Outcome and Assessment Information Set (OASIS), home care, 174–175, 178, 180, 225
Outcome-based quality improvement (OBQI), 171–173, 175, 180–181, 230
  hypothetical report, 178–180, 179i
  implementing, 175–176, 177t, 178
  reports, 176, 178–180, 179i, 182–183, 184, 185i, 186

Outcome criteria, QA, 212
Outcome measure, 164, 173–174

Palliative care, terminally ill, 47, 102, 106
Palliative medicine, 113
Para-professionals
  training needs, 219
  possible demonstration project, 231
Parenteral infusion, home care, 62
Partnership for Long-Term Care Program, 17
Part-time care, definition of, 140, 143
Patient-level predictors, resource consumption, 148–150
Patient outcomes
  definition of, 172
  home health care agencies, 126
  resource consumption, 153–154
Payment types, home visits, 151
Per-hour payment, home health care, 151
Per-visit payment, home health care, 151
Personal assistance services (PAS), 49
Personal emergency response systems, 20
Personal family-worker relationship, 92–93
Physical therapy, and home care, 22, 67
Physician-assisted suicide, 114
Physicians
  and hospice care, 111, 113–114
  home health care involvement, 200–201
  role in home care planning, 66
  role in home care services, 21, 22
Point of service organization (PSO), 124
Postacute care, 8, 45
Predisposing factors, resource consumption, 149, 150
Preferred provider organization (PPO), 124
Primary care management, high risk patients, 192–193
Privacy, view of home, 80
"Private duty services," 119
Private insurance, hospice care reimbursement, 107

Privatization, home health care, 245
Process, criteria, QA, 212
Proprietary agency, home visits, 150, 151, 156
Prospective payment system (PPS)
  discharge impact, 9
  for home health care, 138, 143, 155, 191–192, 243, 246
Provider-initiated approach, QA, 215, 219–221
Provider role, of family in home care, 81, 87–89
Public health nurses, 4
Public policy, and home care, 23–28, 72–73

Quality, definition setting, 212–213
Quality assessment, QA, 213
  approaches, 215–220
  criteria, 214–215
  cycle, 212
  state role in, 221–222
  technology, development of, 231–232
Quality indicator groups (QUIGs), 176, 177t, 179
Quality measure, home care, 170–172, 227–228

Rationalization of care, home health care, 245
Regulatory approach, QA, 215–216, 219
Regulatory issues, home health care agencies, 123
Rescue interventions, home care, 69
Research, home health care, 49–51, 228–229
"Residual" service, home care as, 44
Resource consumption, home care, 139
Respirators, home use, 60
Respite care, 26, 107
Responsibility, systems of in home care, 81
"Rightsizings", home health care, 117
Robert Wood Johnson Foundation, ix, 17

Saunders, Dame Cicely, 103

Index

Severely disabled
 HBPC study, 195–196, 199–200
 TM/HBHC study, 198
Shands HomeCare, challenges survey, 121–124
Shands Hospital, University of Florida, ix
Single-parent households, 20
Skilled nursing facilities, projected expenditures, 241
Skilled nursing services, 39, 42, 43t, 47
"Smart houses," potential in home care, 21
Social Security Disability Insurance, 8
Social supportive services, 45
Social worker, in hospice care, 112
"Spend down," Medicare/Medicaid eligibility, 17, 23
Spouses, as home care workers, 87
St. Christopher's Hospice, Syndeham, England, 103
Staff
 home health care agencies, 122
 home health visits, 151–152
Staff mix, unit of analysis, 147–148
Start of care (SOC), OBQI, 172, 173, 174
Structural criteria, QA, 212, 229
Success strategies, home health care agencies, 126–128
Supportive care, terminally ill, 103, 106
System-level predictors, resource consumption, 148, 152–153

Task approach, funding standards, 96
Task sharer role, of family in home care, 81, 89–90
Tax Equity and Fiscal Responsibility Act of 1982, 9
Tax incentives, long-term care insurance, 24
Team Managed/Hospital Based Home Care (TM/HBHC), 197–200, 198t
Technology
 and future in home care, 20–21

cost of home care, 68–69
 at home, 5–6
 possible demonstration project, 230
Technology-based home care, 59, 60
 policy issues, 72–73
Technology-dependent person, caregiver responsibilities for, 67
Telecommunications technology, in home care, 63, 64
Telephone-triage, 64
Telepractice, 64
Terminally ill. *See also* Hospice
 care of, 101
 HBPC study, 195–196, 196–197
 TM/HBHC study, 198, 199–200
Therapist, home visit, 148
Total hip replacement (THR), NMHHC study, 201, 202
Total joint replacement (TJR), NMHHC study, 201–203
Total knee replacement (TKR), NMHHC study, 201, 202
Total quality management (TQM), 214
Traditional caregivers, loss of, 4
Training, home health care agencies, 122
Treatment plans, family involvement in, 67
Trust, and home care workers, 92, 96

Unit-level expenses, activity-based cost accounting, 128
University of Florida, ix
Utilization outcomes, OBQI, 173

Visiting Nurse Associations, 4
Volunteers, in hospice care, 113

Wald, Florence, 103
Women, as majority of caregivers, 13
Work, at home devalued, 88
Worker-client interaction, home care, 92

Younger disabled persons
 numbers growing, 19
 underinsured, 38

Springer Publishing Company

Geriatric Home Health Care
The Collaboration of Physicians, Nurses, and Social Workers

Philip W. Brickner, MD, *F. Russell Kellogg*, MD,
Anthony J. Lechich, MD, *Roberta Lipsman*, MSSW,
Linda K. Scharer, MUP, Editors

"The number of older persons in our population is growing explosively. The elder boom will be with us for the next 50 years. Unfortunately, our country lacks a coherent policy, and perhaps even a desire, to meet the long-term care needs of the elderly, even though considerable practical experience and scholarly analysis exist. Substantial data are scattered throughout diverse disciplines, including medicine, nursing, gerontology, social services, and the behavioral and biological sciences. However, these resources are poorly understood and assimilated. We hope that the information we have integrated will prove useful in the development of a broad national policy for the aged."

-from the Preface

Drawing on more than 20 years of work in geriatric home health care, the editors of this book share their experiences in creating and managing home health care programs for the frail aged. They have compiled information from diverse disciplines, including medicine, nursing, gerontology, and social services. Important clinical issues, such as functional ability, mental health, and disease and accident prevention, are discussed as well as physician, nurse, and social worker teams; paraprofessional and family supports; and ethical issues and strategies concerning life support decisions.

Four long-term home health care programs are also described, each with a substantial history of success in working through administrative, financial, and bureaucratic problems. This book should be required reading for all professionals working with the elderly in long-term home health care settings.

1997   320pp.   0-8261-9450-8   www.springerpub.com

536 Broadway, New York, NY 10012-3955 • (212) 431-4370 • Fax (212) 941-7842

Springer Publishing Company

Assessing Satisfaction in Health and Long-Term Care
Practical Approaches to Hearing the Voices of Consumers

Robert A. Applebaum, MSW, PhD,
Jane K. Straker, PhD and *Scott M. Geron*, PhD

Drawing from their own research, the authors have created a book that answers the much asked questions about how to assess the satisfaction of health and long-term care recipients successfully.

Designed to be practical in its application, the book includes many examples of questions and approaches used to assess consumer satisfaction. Part I provides an overview in which the authors discuss theories, approaches to measuring consumer satisfaction, and how to implement a consumer data collection strategy. Part II focuses on a broad range of specific areas or settings for assessment including in-home care, nursing homes, and assisted living.

This concise book is a must read for practitioners, researchers, and students committed to listening to the voices of their clients and improving the delivery of care. Helpful web site addresses offer more information on the topics.

Contents:
- Why the Growing Interest in Consumer Satisfaction?
- Theory of Consumer Satisfaction
- Approaches to Measuring Consumer Satisfaction
- Implementing a Consumer Data Collection Strategy
- Measuring Consumer Satisfaction with In-Home Care
- Resident Satisfaction in Nursing Homes and Assisted Living
- Measuring Consumer Satisfaction With Health Care
- Using Consumer Survey Results: Completing the Quality Cycle

1999   152pp.   0-8261-1305-2   *www.springerpub.com*

536 Broadway, New York, NY 10012-3955 • (212) 431-4370 • Fax (212) 941-7842